D0526584

No one should feel scared to tr_____ ... personal stories in Lisa's entertain... ____ ... more people to join the ever-growing running community. I promise you won't regret it.

Nell McAndrew, 2:54:39 marathon runner and author of
Nell McAndrew's Guide to Running

Thank you, Lisa, for this thoroughly enjoyable read. Your book is so full of anecdotes, interesting snippets, humorous moments and some wisdom about our amazing sport that I hardly noticed the time pass on my two-hour flight to Cape Town. Looking forward to volume two!

Bruce Fordyce, nine-time winner of South Africa's
Comrades ultramarathon

This book gives a voice to the many runners who've found salvation, incredible camaraderie, love and laughter through running. The descriptions of the shenanigans and struggles that go on in every race will amuse and amaze you. Your Pace Or Mine? *proves that you don't have to be fast to find running fun.*

Jo Pavey, four-time Olympian and
2014 European Championship gold medallist

Like me, Lisa believes that the world is a community and we need each other. Her tales of the runners she's helped and been helped by during dozens of challenging marathons are incredibly moving.

Lornah Kiplagat, Kenyan-born multiple World Champion
and three-time Olympian

The heartiest recommendation I can give for this glorious book is that having read it, I wanted immediately to go for a run, and to laugh while doing so. An absolute tonic – and a very funny read.

Paul Tonkinson, comedian and *Runner's World* UK columnist

Lisa Jackson has been there and got the running T-shirt, having experienced running highs and lows from every viewpoint. This book takes you on a running rollercoaster of Lisa's experiences and shows you why it's worth the journey.

Liz Yelling, two-time British Olympian and former training partner to Paula Radcliffe

If you ever wanted to run a marathon and didn't think you could, then have-a-go-heroine Lisa Jackson might inspire you to do just that and more! Read it, put your trainers on and 'run the dream' – you'll be a much better person for it.

Rory Coleman, holder of nine Guinness World Records, and veteran of 940 marathons, 235 ultramarathons and 12 Marathon des Sables

Jackson reads like a barefoot romp in the park on a rainy day: refreshing, quirky, deeply insightful, and not afraid to get her feet dirty!

Lorraine Moller, Olympic medallist and Boston Marathon winner

The often hilarious tale of Lisa, an adorable fruitcake of a runner: she's not fast, but she's fun, and behind the interesting hats and colourful gear is a girl of great determination and grit, who turns up marathon after marathon, and gets them done with a smile!

Traviss Willcox, Guinness World Record holder and chairman of the 100 Marathon Club

Lisa's book is a great read! It's not only inspirational but gives practical advice to aspiring marathoners and ultramarathoners.

Jeff Galloway, US Olympian, designer of the Run Walk Run Method

Playfulness and connecting with other runners are key to my approach to running – and to Lisa's, too. Your Pace Or Mine? is a fascinating account of all the fun that can be had on every run once you take the time to engage with the runners around you.

Robert Young aka Marathon Man UK, world record holder (370 marathons/ultras in 365 days, and the 'longest known distance run in history' – 373.75 miles) and winner of the 3,100-mile 2015 Race Across America

In this brilliant book Lisa lays bare, sometimes literally, her life as a runner. She explores the lessons running can teach us all with humour and humility; let her be your guide and get ready to feel inspired and fulfilled with every step you take.

Alison Hamlett, former North Pole Marathon world record holder, 25-time marathon finisher and author of *Need to Know? Running*

A glorious celebration of life on two feet and all we can learn from it. I defy anyone to read this without wanting to grab their trainers, dress up as a fairy, and find a friend to laugh away a run with.

Elizabeth Hufton, editor of *Women's Running* UK

A terrific insight into the strange and strangely beautiful mind of a runner. We've all been there… although most of us have kept our clothes on!

Phil Hewitt, author of *Keep on Running*

A wonderfully written, inspirational and philosophical book, not just about running but also about life and the many challenges it can throw at us. Heartbreakingly sad in some chapters, hilarious in others, it's a great read. Lisa's amazing multiple marathon achievements and the life lessons she has gained make for compelling reading.

Christina Macdonald, launch editor of *Women's Running* UK and author of *Run Yourself Fit*

Lisa's book shows how amazing all of us who run really are: how running can take us to so many places inside ourselves – and around the world. And she really does want everyone to go out and experience some of those runs first hand.

Ultrarunner Pam Reed, veteran of over 100 marathons and eighty 100-milers

Running is the greatest metaphor for life and Lisa's book captures the essence of it beautifully. A must-read!

Elana Meyer, World Champion and Olympic silver medallist

Love it! Whether you are a seasoned racer or nervous newbie you can't help but be inspired by Lisa. Her warm and honest storytelling will have you laughing and gasping in equal measure – and then you'll go out and put your running shoes on, which is what Lisa would want!

Danielle Sellwood, co-founder of Sportsister.com

An inspiring tale that proves that anyone, anywhere, can become a runner.

Rick Pearson, managing editor of *Men's Running* magazine

Lisa's approach to life, marathon running and writing about marathon running is so joyful and infectious, it's impossible to resist. This book will inspire you to run 100 marathons and keep laughing every step of the way.

Rhalou Allerhand, online news editor of *Runner's World* UK

Aimed at motivating absolutely everyone to become passionate about running – without worrying about whether they'll be any good at it – Lisa's inspirational book is sure to start a chat-running craze.

Justine Roberts, founder of Mumsnet and Gransnet

I laughed and I cried along with Lisa as she recounts her journey from non-runner to ultramarathoner. It makes you proud to be part of the same community, and gives you hope of reaching your own personal goals.

Leanne Davies, owner and founder of Run Mummy Run

Since meeting Lisa a decade ago, then reading her first book, Running Made Easy, *and following her progress in her latest book, she's been a complete inspiration. I love the fact that she's a real, normal woman who proves that anything is possible if you want it enough. Thanks to Lisa's enthusiasm and encouragement I'm training for my first (half) marathon!*

Gaby Huddart, editor of *Prima* magazine

Lisa calls running 'the most life-affirming sport', and this zestful romp of a book affirms life on every page. It's funny, wise, and full of vivid stories. Lisa claims to run slowly, but she writes with the spring and verve of a champion.

Roger Robinson, masters marathon champion,
author of *Running in Literature*

An honest, funny and inspiring read that brings a whole new meaning to the term 'running naked'!

Joe Williams, co-founder and director of UKSportsChat

I've always been safe in the knowledge that any struggling runners I see will be scooped up by the wonderful, kind-hearted Lisa Jackson and will make it to the finish line. Now I hear the real stories of what goes on at the back of the pack where people are running with their hearts and not just their feet, I realise how much I've missed. Uplifting, wise and entertaining, this is the only book I've read about running that's made me want to slow down and not speed up!

Juliet McGrattan, GP, runner and health writer

Lisa might not be the fastest marathon runner in the world, or the most competitive, but she has to be one of the funniest. As a fiercely competitive runner myself, she's opened my eyes to the reason why I started running in the first place: running can be fun, something that sporting myopia had made me forget! This book takes you on Lisa's unique journey: you'll laugh, you'll cry and she'll be there every step of the way. She'll even don industrial amounts of Vaseline and run naked: what more could you ask for?

David Castle, editorial director of *Men's Running*

A hilarious yet deeply heart-warming read, this book proves that running is never just about the time you take, it's always also about the journey you've taken.

Tina Chantrey, consultant editor of *Women's Running* UK
and Shewhodaresruns blogger

I absolutely adore Lisa's attitude and approach to running. She seems to look right through all the competitiveness that often surrounds marathons and embraces the pure pleasure of an event where people come together to push through physical limits and celebrate the joy of running.

Julia Buckley, author of *The Fat Burn Revolution*

A truly inspirational read for runners of all levels. I cried, I laughed out loud, and then I couldn't wait to go for a run.

Sally Brown, journalist

YOUR PACE OR MINE?

WHAT RUNNING TAUGHT ME ABOUT LIFE, LAUGHTER AND COMING LAST

LISA JACKSON

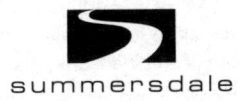

summersdale

YOUR PACE OR MINE?

Summersdale Publishers Ltd
46 West Street
Chichester
West Sussex
PO19 1RP
UK

www.summersdale.com

Printed and bound in the Czech Republic

ISBN: 978-1-84953-827-5

Substantial discounts on bulk quantities of Summersdale books are available to corporations, professional associations and other organisations. For details contact Nicky Douglas by telephone: +44 (0) 1243 756902, fax: +44 (0) 1243 786300 or email: nicky@summersdale.com.

To my mother Leoné Jackson, father Anthony Jackson, and Aunty Rosie and Uncle Ian, who all continue to be an inspiration

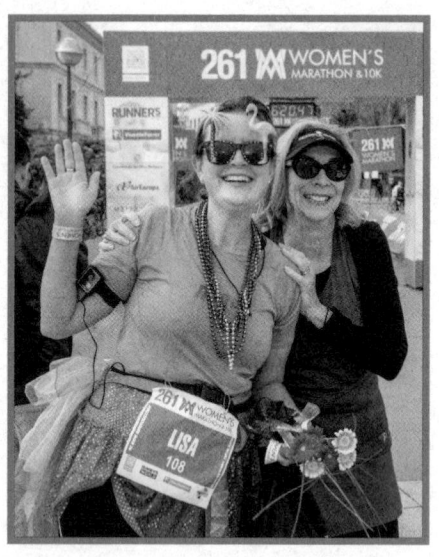

In 1967 Kathrine Switzer was the first woman to officially run the then all-male Boston Marathon. She went on to run 39 marathons (winning the New York City Marathon in 1974) and campaigned to have the women's marathon accepted as an event in the 1984 Olympic Games. The author of three books, she's also an Emmy Award-winning TV marathon commentator and is currently spearheading the 261 Fearless Movement.

Foreword

After running for over 50 years, and considering myself somewhat of a know-it-all about an activity that has been the absolute core of my life, meeting Lisa three years ago opened my eyes to a new look at running. She made it more fun – hilarious, even – and has given me permission not to take myself so seriously. That is more significant than it sounds. It means I – all of us – can embrace the joy without judgement.

This wonderful book isn't about intervals and hill repeats: Lisa doesn't care if you go faster or want to win. She wants you to get out the door. And if wearing a cardboard teapot on your head helps, she regales you with her own experience of doing just that. She doesn't harp on about nutrition either, because anyone who carries a half-pound pack of dates for a mid-race snack has a different agenda. Lisa's agenda is to partake of the best of what running has to offer: connectedness to a community that's wholly egalitarian and encouraging, whether that's a senator trudging alongside you in the rain in the Boston Marathon or a new BFF who's a cancer survivor.

In this book you are swirled into her global running whirlwind as she tackles marathons in cities such as Athens, Paris, Jerusalem and New York. But instead of leaving you breathless, she breathes new air into you: only she can take you from the profundity of death to the ridiculous necessity of Vaseline application when running naked in one emotional roller coaster of a book. Run along with her. Unfailingly generous, Lisa gives you everything she has.

Kathrine Switzer

Contents

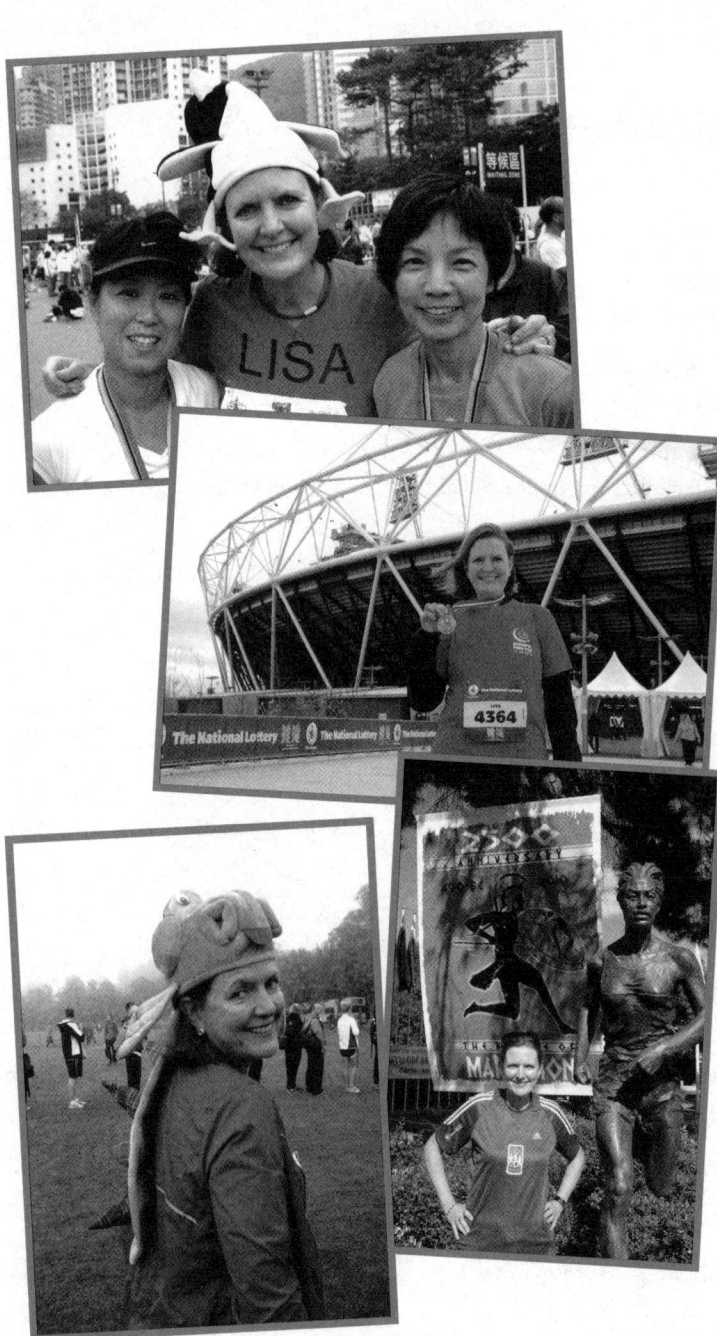

Introduction

> I run. I'm slower than a herd of turtles stampeding through peanut butter, but I run
>
> Bumper sticker

What I'm about to share may come as a bit of a shock to you if you've read my previous how-to-run book, *Running Made Easy*. (And, coming at the start of a book about my passion for running, it might come as a bit of a shock to you even if you haven't!) A lot of the time I wholeheartedly agree with the slogan I once saw on a runner's T-shirt: 'I love running – just not when I'm doing it.'

Looking back, I think I probably should've called my other book *Running Made Easier*, because for me running has never really been easy. No matter how much I've trained or how long I've been doing it, it's always a bit of a struggle. Whether participating in a 5K or 91K, as a woman who had a serious aversion to exercise until the age of 30, there's a huge part of me that thinks I'm crazy. That I'm not cut out for it. That I would rather be sitting on the sofa with a huge glass of ice-cold Sauvignon Blanc than sipping a lukewarm sports drink while chugging up a never-ending highway or gingerly picking my way along a root-riddled trail.

But it's precisely *because* I'm the least likely runner you'll ever meet that running gives me such a thrill. Because I know that even though the winner of a marathon and I have covered exactly the same distance, I've travelled a heck of a lot further to get to the start line, and I don't mean miles. I mean the fact that I've had to surmount being the sort of teenager who snuck to the back of the batting queue in rounders at school just so I wouldn't have to run 50 metres to second base. The sort of person who drove to the corner shop and paid a fortune for parking even though it was only a two-minute walk away. I get an incredible kick out of having decided to reinvent myself as a runner, having chosen to do something so far outside my comfort zone that my new normal is my *discomfort* zone. Even though I more often than not find running a challenge (we're talking 'turtle stampeding through peanut butter' pace here, not speed training, just so you know) I derive an amazing sense of achievement from overcoming the physical and mental difficulty it involves, and from persevering and pushing through. I sincerely hope that by reading my story you'll be tempted to join me and achieve things you too once thought were impossible.

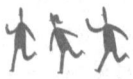

But continually gaining victories over my Inner Sloth isn't the only reason I'm so passionate about running. Some people, like Haruki Murakami, the author of *What I Talk About When I Talk About Running*, run to get away from it all – including their fellow runners. I'm just the opposite. When I run I revel in connecting with other people: fellow slow runners; cheery marshals; poster-toting, you-can-do-it spectators; kids holding out jelly-baby-sticky, high-fiving hands. Stripped of our material possessions, job titles and day-to-day roles, for a few hours we runners are all equal and share a common goal. Our enemy isn't each other, but the distance.

That's why this book, as well as being about my personal running odyssey, includes the stories of those I've stumbled across (or alongside) on the way. I believe that every runner is *equally* amazing. Runners like René on page 198, who didn't let a shattered spine stop him from running 30 marathons in 30 days. Women like Cecy on page 166, a runner with a megawatt smile who runs barefoot to blot out the pain of losing her brother, who was murdered by a Mexican drug gang. Inspirations like Penny on page 67, who stubbornly refused to take up embroidery aged 60 and instead set about running 100 marathons.

I've had a pretty extraordinary journey going from fitness-phobe to UK *Women's Running* magazine's Contributing Editor, one that's involved completing 25 half marathons, 90 marathons and two 91K ultramarathons in 22 different countries on four continents – all in fancy dress. I've dressed up as a zombie, and undressed entirely to run a naked 5K. I've even been an Olympian and crossed the finish line ahead of Usain Bolt in London when, for the first time in the modern Olympics' 116-year history, 5,000 runners were allowed to compete in a five-mile race in the Olympic Stadium before the torch had even been lit.

What have all these many miles taught me? I've learned that by far the hardest part of going after any goal is taking that first wobbly 'what if it doesn't work out?' step. I've learned how the fear of failure is more likely to dash your dreams than trying but failing. I've learned that virtually any challenge becomes downright doable if you focus on having fun (and break it down into bite-size bites and chewable chunks). I've learned that the best way to feel good is to do good. And that death only parts you from your loved ones if you let it: they can be with you in spirit on the start line, the finish line and anywhere in-between. And I've learned that running naked is no big deal – but that failing to apply Vaseline to your inner thighs while doing it most certainly is.

Through countless miles on tarmac, tracks and trails it's been a revelation – and a relief – to realise that you don't have to love *doing* running to love running, at least not all of the time. You don't have to feel like doing it to want to keep doing it. And you certainly don't have to be good at it to succeed. As the self-proclaimed World's Slowest Marathon Correspondent, having come last (yes, last!) in 20 of the marathons I've reported on so far, I've come to the conclusion that running isn't about the time you do, but the time you have while doing it. After reading this book, I'm sure you'll agree.

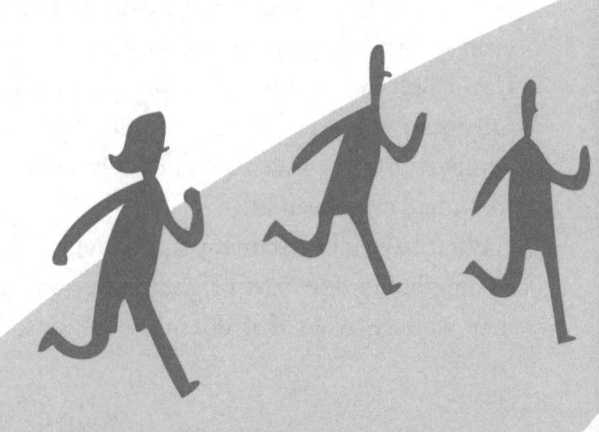

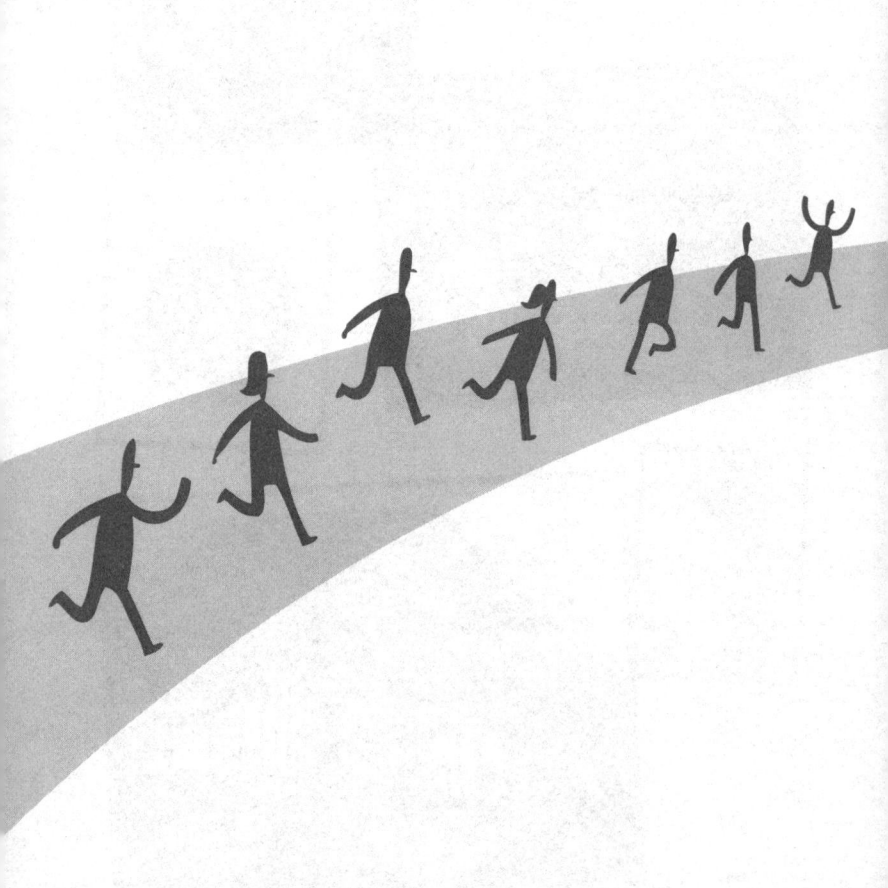

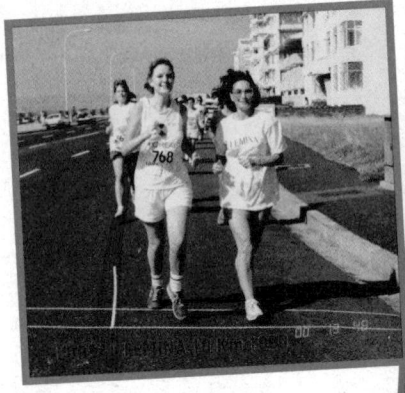
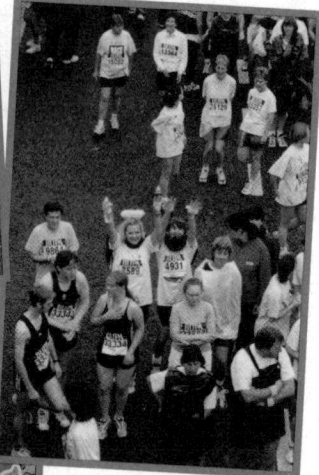
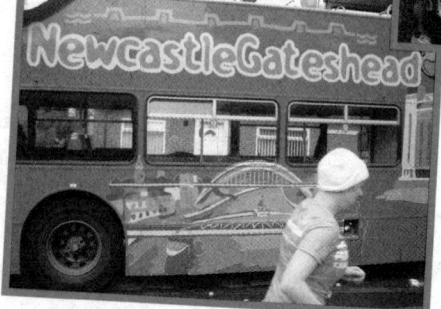
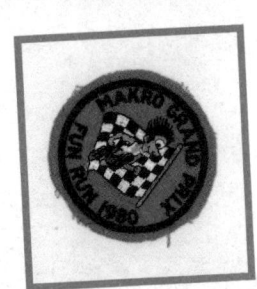
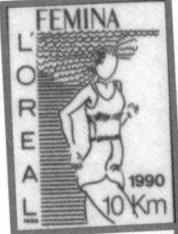
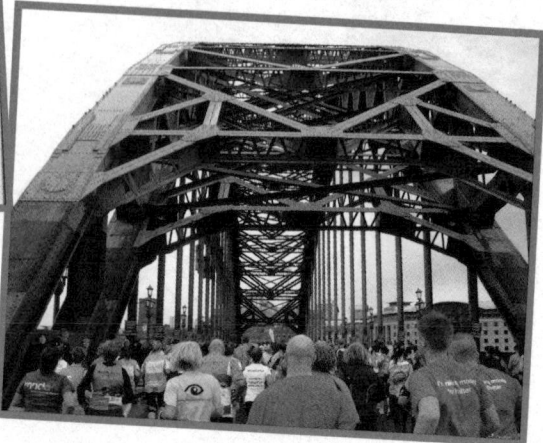

Chapter 1

What running taught me about... taking the first step

> Life leaps like a geyser for those who drill through the rock of inertia
>
> Alexis Carrel

I blame my parents. When asked why I've fallen in love with something I have no chance of ever winning at and that I often find unbelievably difficult, it's the only logical conclusion I can come to. If I hadn't grown up with a Dad who was a national cross-country champion at university, I probably wouldn't be a runner today. And if one of my earliest memories of my mother hadn't been of her running up the steep hill next to our house in Pretoria in South Africa wearing a groovy little Pucci-print miniskirt, I'm sure I'd now spend my spare time swigging wine as a member of a book club, or singing gospel in a choir. Civilised pursuits that don't involve stinky kit, bulk-buying diarrhoea medication or your toenails looking like pork scratchings. But no, I, the world's most unathletic baby, had to go and be born to two activity-addicted parents.

Ever since I'd been given a school report that gave me the worst possible score for 'gross motor co-ordination' and the best possible scores for everything else (I was a six-year-old super-nerd), I'd convinced my parents, myself and everyone around me that I was 'the unathletic one' or 'the academic one', whereas my sister Loren was 'the sporty one'. I'd always associated running with embarrassment and shame – anything but elation. Like many kids, I didn't like doing things I wasn't good at. And boy, I was *always* spectacularly bad at running. I vividly recall break-time at primary school, when our teacher would tell us to run across the football pitch and back. I'd obediently plod along and then turn round, only to see that all my schoolfriends were already back with the teacher, sniggering at me while tucking into their fish-paste sandwiches.

Somehow I found myself, aged 12, running a 5K race around Kyalami, at that time a renowned South African Grand Prix racetrack. I hadn't wanted to go, of course, but my Mum dragged me along. I'd seen Formula One races on TV, so it was strangely thrilling running round the corners that Jody Scheckter, South Africa's 'Wild Man of Motorsport', had hurtled past. I can still remember how awkward running felt then, but also how elated I'd been when I was waved across the finish line, just like a racing car, by a man brandishing a huge black-and-white chequered flag. It was my first taste of the excitement of a big race, but despite my joy at making it round the Kyalami track, it would be ten years before I entered another race.

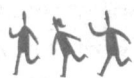

So, back to blaming my parents. My Mum didn't just drag me to my first 5K, she set an example by going for a jog, as she called it, every day. She ran long before the running boom really got off the ground or even before you could readily buy running kit: most people just pulled on a cotton T-shirt, shorts and some uncushioned tennis shoes and that was that. I'm not sure where she got the idea to run in a miniskirt from, but it was the 1970s and glamour was all-important. I wasn't tempted to join my mother – not once. I wasn't envious *at all* of the strange looks she got from our bemused neighbours as she trotted by. I didn't want to be stared at or come home all sweaty or run up the killer hill our house stood at the bottom of.

But my Dad had other ideas. He'd never lost his love of running, and while devoting himself to earning five university degrees and raising a family, he continued to run at least 5K daily, something he does to this day, aged 76. He attributes still being able to fit into his high-school blazer to this little habit he acquired way back when.

My younger sister Loren and I had long ago learned how to trick my Dad – when he used to insist we brush our teeth every evening, we would dutifully troop to the bathroom, thoroughly wet our toothbrushes, place them back in the holder, and then march smugly off to bed, delighted at having outwitted him. So, as a teenager, when my Dad started encouraging us to go for a 2K run each day – and began to check that we'd done so – I knew I could hoodwink him here, too. I'd occasionally shuffle round the block but more often than not I'd get my kit on, leave the house and hide between two parked cars reading a book I'd stuffed up my T-shirt. After 15 minutes I'd sprint the 100 metres home, arriving puffed out enough to convince everyone I'd been for a run.

Years of exercise avoidance followed. I suffered from a phantom case of athlete's foot at high school – for five *years* – so I didn't have to participate in swimming lessons. In my first job on South African *Cosmopolitan* magazine I joined a gym – and went once. I moved to the UK in 1993 at the age of 25. Having joined UK *Cosmopolitan* magazine I adopted a toxic lifestyle of long hours, late-night drinking and eating takeaways standing up on the Tube on the way home. I became so unfit I even struggled to run for the phone, and got breathless walking up a single flight of stairs.

And then, aged 30, one year after I'd begun working for a health magazine called *Zest*, something nothing short of miraculous happened: a colleague persuaded me to enter a 5K Race for Life in Battersea Park and I surprised myself by agreeing to go. 'How hard can it be?' I thought, steadfastly avoiding training and turning up in some flimsy plimsolls I'd swiped off the freebie table at work. Of course, I spent most of the race walking, and when I did run, each step thudded onto the road, sending a shockwave up my leg to my more-than-ample bottom. Running was infinitely harder, and more unpleasant, than I ever remembered. Who likes the sound of their butt flicking the tops of their thighs? Who enjoys having a face the colour of a stop sign? And yet I rushed home afterwards high as a kite, eager to tell my husband Graham about it. Because what had blown me away about the event wasn't the running itself – at that stage it was way too hard to like, even for a few steps – it was the *atmosphere*. Hundreds of partners, husbands and friends had turned out to cheer us, and I remember being very moved by the sight of several dads under a tree jigging babies on their hips while swilling champagne and guarding a giant pile of kitbags.

I got chatting to a group of women who were all doing the race for loved ones affected by cancer. As they told their stories I could barely see where I was going, my vision was so blurred by tears. Far from being *competitive* with one another, these women were *collaborative*, turning round to shout encouragement at other participants, urging them to keep going. I didn't learn anyone's name that day but I did get reminded, once again, that running didn't have to mean feeling like a loser, even if you did finish at the back. I also realised that while running really was hard, and involved unimaginable amounts of huffing and puffing, jiggling and wobbling, it also resulted in unimaginable amounts of joy once you'd done it. And when they gave me my medal, well, that was it. I didn't comprehend it then, but they had me. They had me for life. That night I started a tradition I've kept up ever since – I went to sleep wearing it.

By 1998 my aunt Rosemary, my Dad's sister who lived in Oxford with her British husband Ian, had already spent five years trying to persuade me to run a 10K with her. Aunty Rosie had a not-so-secret ambition of turning me into her running partner. One of the first things she'd said to me when I'd arrived in England was, 'Are you still running?' I'm sure she knew full well I'd never started running but she continued to nag me gently to enter a race with her. In the end it wasn't pester power that won the day, or even the fantastic time I had at the charity 5K, but all-consuming envy. My aunt announced that she'd got a place in the Great North Run, at that time the world's biggest half marathon.

'Noooooo!' I thought. 'Aunty Rosie's almost double my age and now she's going to be able to say she's run a half *marathon*!' The word 'marathon', even though it was preceded by the word 'half', sounded impressively, impossibly far.

That very day I posted off my race application, half of me hoping that I'd left it so late I wouldn't get in. But fate had other ideas. Just a few weeks later a letter arrived in the post. I had been given a place. I remember jumping into the air, punching my fists ceilingwards, but even before my feet hit the floor a terrible realisation hit me: I'd actually have to run 21K. Over 13 miles. A scary 16K longer than my red-faced Race for Life. What now? In the age before Google I rushed to consult a running-mad colleague.

'How do I find out how to train for a half marathon?' I asked *Zest*'s Deputy Editor Sally Brown.

'*Runner's World*,' she replied sagely. 'Try reading *Runner's World*.'

Wow, there was actually a whole magazine dedicated to running? Who knew? And so it was that I became *Runner's World*'s No 1 fan, stalkerish in my desire to pick up every shred, scrap and crumb of knowledge that would help me attain my new goal. I read every single word, starting from the Editor's letter all the way through to the Classifieds in the back. I even read all the dozens of advertising leaflets and flyers that came with it. And by the time I'd finished I felt I knew every staff member personally. To me they were the Rock Gods of Running. I knew their times, I knew the last race they'd run, I knew what they ate for breakfast.

Nick Troop particularly endeared himself to me when he wrote in his Publisher's letter about his newfound respect for runners at the back of the pack. As a runner capable of doing a marathon in under four hours (the benchmark for officially being called 'speedy'), he'd once been asked to pace runners aiming to finish in under six hours and had been amazed at how difficult he'd found it. He cited spending over two hours longer on his feet as the main reason for the agony he suffered – and had been full of praise for the tortoises he'd until then tended to dismiss as not having made as much effort as the front runners. 'Slow runners, I salute you!' was his humble apology. I was utterly amazed and very moved that a fast runner had taken the time to acknowledge that we runners at the back of the pack deserved praise just as much – if not more so – than our fleeter-footed friends.

My favourite page in *Runner's World* was The Penguin Chronicles written by John 'The Penguin' Bingham who, as a 43-year-old, 240-lb (109-kg) smoker, had taken the plunge and morphed into a slow runner with the catchphrase 'Waddle on, friends'. One column particularly touched me. In it, The Penguin described running a marathon next to a 40-something man who had tears streaming down his face. When asked why he was crying the runner, who'd already told The Penguin how he'd always worked hard, raised a family and done all the things he thought he should do, had replied: 'Because... I just realised that in my entire life, no one has ever cheered for me before.' At that, The Penguin, too, had started to cry.

Every time I re-read that story I couldn't help but well up. Because I knew exactly what he meant. The fact that people who didn't know you wanted you to achieve your goal – and were prepared to shout themselves hoarse to let you know that – was almost unbearably moving. It was the exact feeling of uplift and gratitude I'd felt while running the Race for Life. Like the crying marathoner, I too had done all the things I'd believed were expected of me: excelling at school, being a dutiful daughter and a super-conscientious employee. And yet no one had cheered. Now I had the chance to be cheered – all I had to do was run more than twice as far as I'd ever done before. The thought terrified me.

Fuelled by fear I embarked on *Runner's World*'s half-marathon training plan. Fortunately, Day One involved only one thing: Rest. 'Oh good,' I thought, 'I'm going to do just fine as I'm *exceedingly* good at resting.' Day Two was heaps more challenging than Day One, as I actually had to do some running. Without the distractions of chatting and cheering that I'd had in my 5K, I focused on what was happening to my body, and it wasn't pretty. I was plagued by chafing – my knees would rub together until they were raw, and when later I swapped from shorts to cotton trousers the constant friction between my thighs created holes in the fabric. It would be years before I discovered the deep joy of Lycra capris.

Having found my ideal time to run – during a section of my commute home from central London – the days turned into weeks and I was relieved to notice that after a while my bottom stopped jellying about and I was able to run ever-increasing distances without searching for the nearest park bench to sit on and catch my breath.

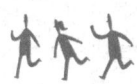

That autumn Aunty Rosie and I travelled up to Newcastle-upon-Tyne for the Great North Run. On race day I liberally dusted myself with glitter, intending to run dressed as the famed Tyne and Wear landmark, the *Angel of the North*, Antony Gormley's stunning 20-metre-tall steel sculpture with a 54-metre wingspan. The event couldn't have been more of a 'Wow' if they'd attached feathered showgirl headdresses to each of the 50,000 runners taking part. As we surged over the iconic Tyne Bridge the Red Arrows aerobatic display team screeched overhead, trailing patriotic red, white and blue smoke, causing me to look up and lose my feathered halo. Although I was more than happy to continue running in just my angel wings, Aunty Rosie darted backwards, frantically scrabbling for the halo and triumphantly retrieving it. In the process she almost caused the running equivalent of a motorway pile-up: the air turned even bluer as dozens of angry runners blurted out expletives while trying to dodge her.

Undaunted we pressed on, revelling in the crowd's rapturous cheering, doing disco-dancing moves every time we encountered a band belting out a pop song, chanting 'Oggi, oggi, oggi! Oi, oi, oi!' with utter delight as we passed through the underpasses. But our jollity turned to dismay when, as the minutes ticked by, it grew colder and colder and started to rain. Being half-marathon virgins we'd dressed in T-shirts and hadn't brought along running jackets. We simply hadn't accounted for how temperamental the British weather can be. We tried to ignore the cold and rain and focus on the pot-banging spectators and grinning kids in South Shields for the final few miles, but had to resort to running with our hands tucked in our armpits to keep them warm.

Our second schoolgirl error was not bringing any food. We'd assumed there'd be plenty of snacks, or at least sports drinks, along the route, but I don't recall being offered any at all. We both started to feel slightly faint, so when a spectator stepped forward with a cardboard box full of race refreshments we eagerly ran over to grab some to boost our blood sugar. Unfortunately, the kind stranger had obviously assumed we'd be running on a hot and sunny day and had, therefore, thoughtfully stocked up on ice lollies to help cool us down. With chattering teeth, we each forced one down, despite the fact that they made us feel even more frigid than we had before.

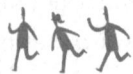

Eventually, after interminable hills and a short, sharp downhill section that made many of us yelp in pain, we were on the home straight. Running beside the sleet-dusted North Sea we experienced a growing sense of disbelief. We'd made it. We had actually run half of that most magical of distances, a marathon. Crossing the finish line with our stopwatches reading 2h55, my aunt, her chin blue with cold, gave me a huge hug. Then, like two tipsy old ladies who'd gone a little overboard with the sherry, we hung onto each other for dear life as we zigzagged over to a charity tent to warm up. Having eagerly wriggled out of our sopping wet clothes and pulled on dry ones, we tucked into a huge portion of steaming-hot, vinegary chips. Paradise on a paper plate.

On the top deck of the double-decker bus that transported us from the finish back into the town centre, Aunty Rosie and I stared out of the window. As the miles rolled by it dawned on us – we'd actually *run* all of this. Yes, on our own two feet we'd covered a distance that was taking absolute ages to traverse by bus. We were now 'real' runners. We wanted to open a window and shout this astonishing news to anyone who'd listen. The hypothermia and hypoglycaemia were already distant memories because all we could think of, as we lovingly stroked our medals, was 'What's next?'

So what did running teach me about getting started? I learned that the longest journey really does begin with a single step (even if that step is taken in plimsolls). But that that single step is, in all likelihood, the hardest you'll ever take. It taught me that with *any* project or ambition it's best not to overthink things, something my political-analyst husband catchily calls 'analysis paralysis', but just to jump in feet first and see how things pan out. If I'd waited till I was properly trained and owned the right trainers to enter Race for Life I probably wouldn't be a runner today. The secret to getting started? St Francis of Assisi summed it up perfectly: 'Start by doing what is necessary. Then do what is possible. And suddenly you're doing the impossible.'

'How I took my first steps'

'I didn't think I could run – but I've now done 12 marathons'

I was never very sporty at school, mainly due to having Clumsy Child Syndrome: hockey, tennis and netball were all very hard for me due to my poor hand-eye co-ordination. The first time I ran round the block I found it incredibly difficult: I could hardly breathe and got a massive stitch. I

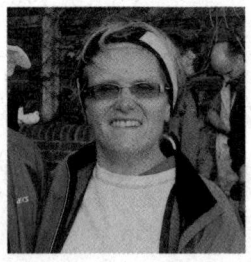

remember thinking, 'What on earth am I doing?' But then I spoke to my Dad, who's a runner, and he told me I could prevent stitches by breathing deeply. So I kept on going, mainly because I'm very stubborn and wanted to show that I could do it, and gradually everything got a bit easier. My first race was a 5K Race for Life in 2003, which I completed with my four-year-old nephew Jack. I loved the festive atmosphere and have marshalled or participated ever since.

My favourite kind of running is cross-country: running through woods is lovely, and the scenery changes during the seasons (I even like ploughing through thigh-deep snow). I live in Croydon in south London which is more famous for its 1960s high-rise buildings than its open spaces, but since I've been running with Striders of Croydon, I've discovered some lovely routes through parks, fields and forests. I may be one of the slower runners, but I love encouraging anyone who's new to the club because I valued the support I got when I became a member. Having completed 12 marathons in 12 years I now dream of joining the 100 Marathon Club and doing the 156-mile Marathon des Sables, which I can't quite believe as I'm someone who never thought I could run a single step.

Victoria Legge, 45, Croydon, London, England

'I always thought running was for "real runners"'

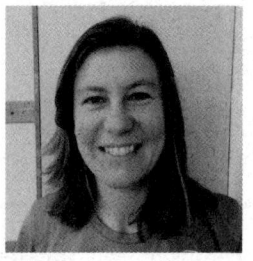

Running means so much to me because I never thought I'd be able to do it. It never even occurred to me I could be a runner – it was as if runners were a whole different species. When I ran alongside Lisa in the Barcelona Marathon I hadn't entered the race – I'd simply come to encourage the runners from the sidelines. I could see Lisa was struggling so I offered to keep her company and trotted alongside her as best I could, wearing jeans and carrying a handbag.

I'd started my love affair with running just six months before, but it was the first time I'd watched a marathon and I was desperately thrilled and attracted to it all. I'm a mum of three and found it hard to find the time to go to the gym so I started running for 20 minutes three times a week but didn't actually enjoy it. To help me get out of bed early and go for a run I'd write RMYFGFTWD on my hand the night before: it stood for 'Running makes you feel good for the whole day'. Then one morning I had an itch to go further and ran to and from my mother-in-law's house 20 minutes away. I experienced an incredible euphoria from actually reaching a place under my own steam. After that I started planning routes on milermeter.com and running to places I loved in Barcelona.

During the marathon Lisa told me that she'd also found running really difficult to start with and suggested I do a half marathon as that would give me a goal. I only ran 2K with her but that conversation stayed with me and a year later I did it. Now I've set my sights on next year's Barcelona Marathon. I can't quite believe I'm actually a 'real' runner now.

Clare Butler, 40, Barcelona, Spain

'I was so overweight I could barely walk when I took the decision to become a runner'

By the time I got to the age of 49 I was so overweight I could barely walk, so I felt I had no choice but to lose weight. Quite early in the journey I met Lisa and decided I wanted to run a 5K as she kept raving about how much fun they were. My first walk/run training session was a tremendous struggle due to my weight, but on race day I puffed and panted until eventually I crossed the finish line and felt elated as my first medal was hung around my neck.

I did my second 5K with Lisa and she got me through by promising me walk breaks and running in front of me calling my name. By the end I think everyone on the course knew who I was! I got my own back, though, as I persuaded her to do a 50K cycling event in hilly Sussex. This time I was in front shouting for her to keep up with me. At the final rest stop I had to drag Lisa back onto the bike as she wanted to stay and eat cakes, but with a little encouragement she did get back in the saddle and we completed the race.

Next I attempted triathlons – the one at Hever Castle had a hill so steep that I was forced to go so slowly I ended up falling off my bike into a ditch.

I promised Lisa I'd do a marathon with her but I've recently been diagnosed with cancer. I may not be able to run at the moment but there are wheelchair races so David Weir, watch out! I'm going to ask Lisa to hire one and do it with me!

Lyndall Melvyn, 54, London, England

Sadly, Lyndall died before she could run a marathon with me – this is one of my greatest regrets as I know she and I would've laughed through and loved every second of it.

'I learned you don't have to be fast to take up running'

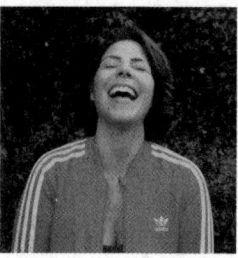

I am not the sporty type. As a child I briefly dabbled in dance; at secondary school I half-heartedly played netball (and was always goalie as it entailed the least effort); and then in my late 20s I intermittently took the odd gym class. That was the extent of my exercise regime when I undertook my first run, aged 33. By that time, I was a single mum to a feisty two-year-old who seemed doggedly determined that I should be deprived of any shut-eye, and I hadn't exercised in a couple of years. Given my tiredness, and my predisposition to laziness (sloth being my go-to mode), I never would have considered taking up running were it not for my new job. Or, more precisely, my new colleague, Lisa. She gently cajoled me into joining her and her merry bunch of lunchtime runners, saying something like: 'Just try it. If you don't like it, you never have to do it again.' But I did like it. On that first run Lisa taught me how to find a comfy pace, dispelling my total misconception that you have to be fast to take up running; with practice you can become that way, but you can start as slow as you like – I'd never thought of that. She also taught me not to worry about the hordes of passers-by while legging it around London in Lycra. The best bit, however, was the good feeling at the end, a mixture of pride and achievement.

Sadly, after a while Lisa left the company. I carried on running twice a week until I left, too. Running has since gone in two-year cycles for me. Currently, I'm getting back into it again, but with this being my third stint I know *exactly* how to be a runner: you just get out there and do it.

Tara Nathanson, 41, Falmouth, England

'I went from obese smoker to ultrarunner'

I was sporty until the age of 14 – and then did no exercise till I was 35 for a variety of reasons: going to boarding school, not having anyone to motivate me and starting to smoke, drink and eat junk food. Then, one day in 2011, for no reason other than wanting to get out of the house, 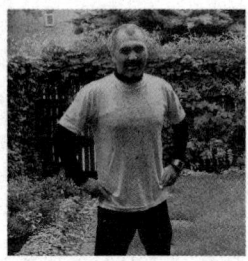 I went for a run. It was rather painful as I was obese, but I was surprised to find I rather liked it. I ran a very sweaty 7K that day, but made frequent rest stops. The next day I went for a 5K run and already found it easier. Within a week I was running non-stop for 10 to 15 minutes and began going out regularly. I didn't enjoy the insults about my size that guys shouted from their vans but got round that by using earphones.

I was smoking ten cigarettes a day then, so when I did my first ten-mile race seven months later, I just couldn't stop coughing at the finish. After that I cut down to just a couple a day and drank less too (until then I'd been having up to 30 units a week). I surprised myself by completing three 10Ks, two half marathons and two ten-milers in my first year.

Then the Facebook ultrarunning community tempted me to enter an ultra. I did day one of the Vanguard Way Ultra and finished fifth. Since then I've done 15 ultras ranging from 80K to 160K. Along the way I've lost 10 kg and, on New Year's Day 2014, having smoked for 23 years, I quit completely. From barely being able to run for two minutes it's truly amazing to think I can now run non-stop for nine hours.

Özgur Gülec, 39, Croydon, London, England

Having done a few marathons in my 30s I became a lapsed runner. Turning up for a 5K parkrun shocked me back into action, however, as I managed just one 2.5K lap before retiring. Soon afterwards I joined a running club with a friend. Neither of us was brave enough to turn up solo as we both erroneously thought clubs were only for fast runners. I used to hang out with Lisa at the back of the slow group, but each week I tried to run further up the field. I now lead the group and love encouraging and having a mid-run chat with different people. The biggest challenge I've faced so far? Wearing leggings in winter. It seems quite normal now – in fact, the louder the gear the better!

Tony Flowers, 45, Croydon, London, England

Thinking back, I hated every minute of my first run. My legs were heavy, I couldn't control my breathing, and I couldn't keep up with the pack. But I started making progress and that motivated me. I learned to persevere and be patient – even when injuries set me back. Running has transformed my life: I've made friends with lots of interesting people and I've lost weight. Most importantly, I now realise I'm capable of doing more than I ever thought. I've even managed to do a marathon. When Lisa, whose running camp I went on, invited me to do the Bacchus Marathon I initially chickened out but reconsidered. My goal was to finish... alive! And I'm rather surprised to report I actually did. Who knows, maybe there'll be another in the future.

Andrea Rinaldi, 36, Renfrewshire, Scotland

I'm not a runner, not yet anyway. At the age of 28 I went from working towards my first 10K to having a blood clot in my leg and being diagnosed with asthma. I spent the next few months in a wheelchair followed by some time on crutches and finally, in the past year, I've been focusing on getting my fitness back. Having learned to use the treadmill at the gym I found it a bit disheartening when my 80-year-old gym buddy could walk faster and further than me. But I persisted and can now walk for ten minutes and run for one. My 10K may be a long way off but I no longer fear that it won't happen.

Sarah Halpin, 29, Ireland

I reviewed Lisa's book, *Running Made Easy*, back in 2004 when working on a local newspaper in Croydon and it inspired me to try her 5K plan. I recall feeling like a superhero after my first 16-minute walk/run shuffle one dark winter's night, pretty much the way I felt recently after giving birth to my first child. Having run half marathons since, the pride I felt in completing those 16 minutes seems a little silly now, but at the time I might as well have summited Mount Everest. I got hooked on the feeling of *having been* running: initially I wasn't overly fond of the actual running, preferring the intense afterglow, which was definitely worth the slog. Somewhere along the way I began to enjoy running itself, and now I genuinely love it.

Laura Greaves, 34, Sydney, Australia

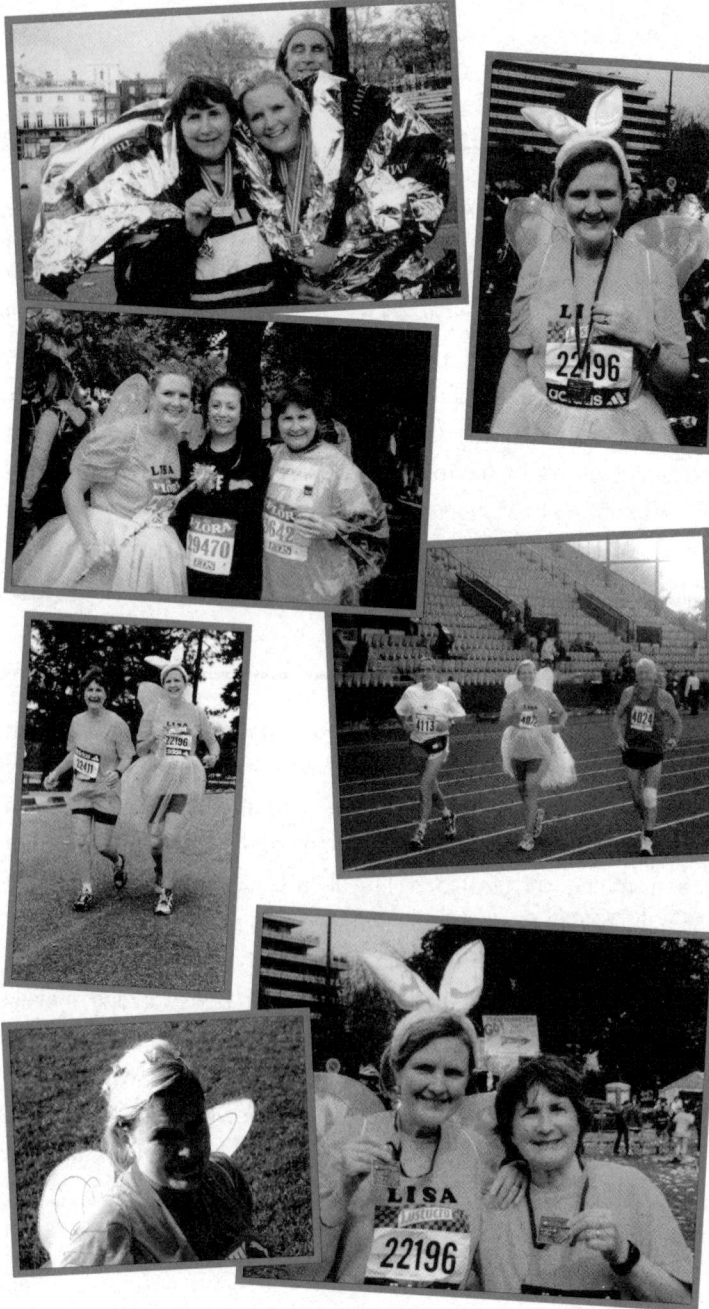

Chapter 2

What running taught me about... fear

As a child my parents strictly forbade me to use the f-word, and to this day I wince whenever I hear someone say it. But now, as I hurtle towards my fifties, I know there's another four-letter f-word that's far, far worse, and yet, when you're growing up, no one warns you about. That word is fear. I love the motivational saying that claims it stands for False Expectations Appearing Real – how many times do we let anticipated failures and imagined disasters stand in the way of us chasing our dreams? As the American author Mark Twain so humorously put it: 'I have been through some terrible things in my life, some of which actually happened.' Fear is the reason so many of us lead lives full of regret about what should have or could have been. And fear is the reason many people never take up running even though, deep down, they know they want to.

Having overcome my fear of failing to finish a half marathon, I knew I couldn't let fear stop me taking the next step: running a marathon. But I knew the marathon I chose couldn't be just any old marathon. As I suspected it would be the only 26.2 miles I'd ever run, it simply had to be the best. 'Go large or go home,' my sister Loren said. It would have to be the London Marathon, despite the fact that it was harder to get into than a two-sizes-too-small corset – I knew because Aunty Rosie had tried no fewer than six times without success. Once again, my *Zest* magazine colleague Sally came to the rescue. In November she told me I could have the media place she could no longer use due to an injury. I couldn't believe my luck, and promised to help Aunty Rosie secure a place by fundraising for charity.

When I told my Dad that I was going to run a marathon his first reaction, based on the fact I was 3 st (19 kg) overweight, was: 'Do you think that's a good idea, my lovey?'

'Dad, I've never wanted to do anything more in my whole life,' I replied passionately.

'Well, you do know you're risking kidney failure,' he warned. I was horrified, as I couldn't recall reading that running causes kidney damage, but nonetheless I remained steadfast in my resolve.

'It's a risk I'm willing to take,' I said firmly.

'Well, just don't overdo it,' he said. Putting down the phone, I immediately researched renal failure in runners and was relieved to find that it was unlikely unless you were under-trained and severely dehydrated, and had taken nonsteroidal anti-inflammatory drugs such as ibuprofen – all of which I resolved not to do.

With our marathon places assured, all that stood between us and the start line was some fundraising (old-fashioned sponsorship forms took care of that) and, of course, some training. The latter was a heck of a lot more daunting than the former, but once again *Runner's World* came to the rescue with a doable programme that I suspected I might just about manage. And during a water-cooler moment I managed to persuade a fellow *Zest* colleague, Alex, to fill the magazine's second media-place slot.

Several times a week for three-and-a-half long months Alex and I dutifully headed down to The Embankment after work to train. My husband Graham had been temporarily posted to Bahrain so I could devote myself wholeheartedly to my marathon preparation. Alex was great company so I soon honed the chat-run technique that would serve me so well in the years to come. *Runner's World* had informed me of the famous 'talk test': if you aren't able to talk, you're overdoing it, but if you're able to sing, you're not running hard enough. We took training very seriously, jokingly aiming for at least 10,000 words a minute. I often thought of Alan Sillitoe's brilliant short story, *The Loneliness of the Long-Distance Runner*. For Alex and me, *The Chattiness* would've been more apt.

We also made sure we stretched religiously. One evening we decided to do our stretches at the bottom of the Duke of York Steps on The Mall. During one deltoid stretch – the one where you extend an arm across your body and use the forearm of your other arm to pull it closer to your chest – we were approached by a group of Japanese tourists who stood staring at us for a few moments before, rather solemnly, walking over to shake our outstretched hands. 'Nice to meet you,' they said smiling and bowing. Had they mistaken us for a welcoming committee from Buckingham Palace just up the road? Did they think we were street performers pretending to be living statues? We didn't know then, and I guess we'll never know. Looking at each other in amazement, we responded in the only way that seemed appropriate at the time. We politely bowed back.

Another odd episode occurred in Kensington Gardens one Sunday when I was speed-training. Midway through one of the sprint sessions I was accosted by a young woman: 'Excuse me for interrupting your walk,' she said, 'but I wondered if you'd like to learn more about Jesus by coming to church with me this afternoon?'

'My *walk*?' I spluttered. 'I'm in the middle of a *speed* session!' I was too indignant to say any more, and to prove my point turned on my heels and waddled off (a whole lot faster than I'd been training before).

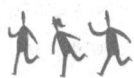

The Thursday before race day Alex and I boarded the Docklands Light Railway from central London to the London Arena to fetch our race numbers. Unusually for avert-your-eyes Londoners, for whom talking to a stranger is tantamount to publicly declaring that you should be sectioned, everyone was chatting happily about their race history and ambitions for the big day. The convivial atmosphere aboard this toy train on stilts as it threaded through east London's skyscrapers was reminiscent of geography field trips at school; I almost expected us all to burst into a rendition of 'If you're happy and you know it, clap your hands!' I felt a warm glow of happiness. I was part of this. I wasn't just here as a supporter. I was here to run. The Marathon. Myself. Lisa, The Non-Sporty One, was a Marathon Runner. A Real Runner. And oh, it felt good.

Walking into the Expo and hearing Ron Goodwin's famous London Marathon music (composed for the film *The Trap*) playing on continual loop fuelled my excitement at seeing the vast number of stalls selling every conceivable running gadget and gizmo. Like a kid at a pick 'n' mix I had no idea where to start. Should I fondle the trainers and inhale their intoxicating new-shoe smell or stand in line for a paper shot glass full of neon-coloured goodness-knows-what? Barge my way into the melee surrounding the bargain bins of sport socks or pluck up the courage to visit the Rock Gods of Running at the *Runner's World* stand? I decided to fetch my race number first.

'Good luck,' beamed the woman who handed me the envelope containing my number and timing chip. 'Enjoy every second because, although you may run many more marathons, you can never run a first one ever again.'

The admin out of the way, I spent the next few hours shopping like Imelda Marcos at a Jimmy Choo buy-one-get-five-free sale. A new water bottle? I just had to have that. Ditto new socks. And laces. And a snack belt. And a strangely jockstrap-like knee bra. And countless leaflets advertising marathons I knew I'd never run. And then I made the mistake of visiting a sports-drink stand, where the salesman asked me about my pre-race nutrition.

'Oh, I've been carbo-loading by eating pasta for dinner twice this week,' I said breezily.

'Is that *all*?' he spluttered. 'That's *never* going to get you round 26.2 miles!'

My heart froze with fear. I pictured myself hitting the dreaded Wall I'd heard so much about like a wrecking ball slamming into a derelict building. I could visualise my legs turning to jelly-and-custard, all my energy draining away like a car whose owner had left its lights on. 'What to do?' I wailed inwardly.

'Basically you should've been eating *tons* of carbs at *every* meal,' he said, 'and of course drinking nothing but sports drink for the past week.'

'What if I start right now, would that do it?' I pleaded.

'I can't say for sure, but you could give it a go.'

I loaded up my by-now-bulging rucksack with as much sports drink as I could carry and staggered around the rest of the Expo like a Marine setting off on a 60-mile swamp yomp, furiously sipping sports drink as I went. I looked around desperately: was there *anything* else, anything at all, that I could buy or do that would get me round on race day? Besides a towelling wristband to mop up the sweat that would be running down my arms (needless to say, I bought two) and a sports watch that cost more than my monthly mortgage (at least here I resisted and reluctantly put it back on the shelf)?

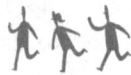

They say you never forget your first time, and they're right. 18 April 1999. Over 16 years later, I can still recall the exact date of my first marathon. My running companions Aunty Rosie and Alex came to stay the night before and, needless to say, I didn't sleep a wink. But *Runner's World* had told me this was normal, and that what was important was to get a good night's rest 'the night before the night before', which I'd dutifully done. Saturday night was a flurry of general panic: 'Oh nooooo! I've lost my race number! No I haven't. It's here. Where's my T-shirt? I've left it at home, I'm sure of it. Can I borrow one? Yes? Phew! Wait, I found it!' Throwing three marathon virgins into the same room the night before their first marathon and expecting them not to get their running tights in a twist is like feeding a toddler neat cola and hoping it'll put her to sleep.

At last, race day dawned and we rose at sparrow's fart to make our way to the start in Greenwich Park. The scene at East Croydon station resembled a zombie movie as slowly, from every direction, runners emerged from the quiet, slowly lightening streets clutching the baggage bags issued at the Expo. As we all piled onto the first train to London Bridge station there was a buzz of excitement. All hell broke loose when we got to London Bridge, however, where the platforms were choked with runners all trying to cram into the overflowing carriages. We looked at each other in dismay – we'd known running the marathon was going to be a challenge, but we didn't expect getting to the start to be.

As yet another packed train drew up alongside us my 59-year-old aunt shouted: 'Out of the way please, make way for the elderly runner!' As the other passengers stepped aside she grabbed our hands and hissed: 'Quick, get on, get on, it's our only chance.' Barging onto the carriage, we tried not to make eye contact with anyone, as we were well aware my aunt looked anything but elderly.

Once off the train, we streamed into Greenwich Park and up a path leading to the Royal Observatory. The hill was very steep and I was soon breathless, which added to my increasing agitation. If I couldn't make it up a short incline without sounding like a nuisance caller, how on earth was I going to run 26.2 miles?

Having located the baggage buses that would transport the bags with our clothes to change into afterwards to the finish line on The Mall, there was a last-minute scramble to get ready. Ever since I'd played the role of the Queen of the Fairies in nursery school I'd dreamed of being a fairy again, so I'd decided that for my one and only marathon I'd once again don a tutu and fairy wings. I also made myself a Blue Peter-esque wand using a giant tube filled with jellybeans and decorated with tinsel. Cicely Mary Barker, whose Flower Fairies books had enchanted me as a child, would've pranced with joy. However, the *pièce de résistance* was my pink T-shirt. When I'd asked my colleague Sally for her most important tip for London, she'd urged me to get my name printed on my T-shirt. 'You'll get twice as much support that way.' By now I knew it was best to heed Sally The Running Guru's advice and so I'd paid to have my name emblazoned across my chest in the biggest, boldest black letters possible.

It took us – the slowest runners and those running for charity – an incredible 17 minutes from when the gun went off to shuffle to the start line, so I had plenty of time to experience the full impact of the tidal waves of fear that washed over me. I couldn't help but replay my Dad's dire warnings about kidney failure over and over in my mind. Still, I distinctly remember thinking that nothing I'd ever set my heart on had mattered to me more. And, melodramatic as it may sound, I thought that if I died that day I would die achieving the greatest goal I'd ever set for myself.

I got more and more nervous until I was sure I was going to be physically sick. But then I remembered an amusing Chinese proverb: 'Unhelpful thoughts are like birds – you might not be able to stop them from crapping on your head but you can stop them from nesting in your hair.' So I decided to kick out the vile vultures and swerve my thoughts away from the subject of Death By Running. Instead I decided to focus on the crazy costumes of those around me – and boy, did I have a lot to choose from. Among them was a man 'sitting' on a toilet (with two fake foam legs dangling in front of him), two people in giant pirate outfits and even a tidy of Wombles (I'm sure that's the collective noun). In fact, no one looked as if they were about to run a marathon, one of the toughest challenges on the planet. They looked as if they'd bought tickets to Comic Con.

Reassured by the fact that I was among like-minded runners, I felt a surge of elation as we finally crossed under the start-line arch and headed off. And then, just 200 metres after setting out, I suddenly found I couldn't breathe. I was faced with something that, no matter how many miles I'd run, I could not have trained for. It was something I'd never seen before and haven't seen since: a long line of male runners with their backs to us, all peeing in unison on the side of the road. Now, I have seen men urinating before, but what had sent a ripple of howling laughter through the entire marathon pack was the fact that one of the runners was a rhino, who was holding his horned head in one hand and his winky in the other. Giddy with a cocktail of every stress hormone known to science coursing through my veins, I thought this was the funniest thing I'd ever, ever witnessed. I laughed so hard that I actually had to stop to get my breath back.

At this point Alex, who was even more nervous than I was, shot off, never to be seen again. Aunty Rosie stuck by me, however, and together we chat-ran through Blackheath, Woolwich and Greenwich. We were utterly blown away by the spectators lining both sides of the road, often several people deep. It really was like running the gauntlet, but instead of having to endure a cacophony of sneers we were treated to a tribute of cheers.

Just after six miles (9.7K) we reached the *Cutty Sark*, the legendary tea clipper. The crowds here were the most boisterous on the entire course and when they saw my outfit they went completely bonkers. You'd think they'd never seen a plump little fairy before. Every inch of my skin was covered in goosebumps as I looped round the ship, and I felt as if I was crowd-surfing as the cheers carried me round. 'This is what Madonna must feel like,' I thought, suddenly becoming aware of how much my jaw was aching from grinning at being treated like a world-class celebrity.

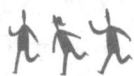

Sadly, my euphoria was short-lived. During training I'd developed a knee niggle and it was now beginning to feel more like a kneecapping. I had no option but to urge my aunt to go on ahead of me. I thought I'd be devastated if I had to run on my own, but the fancy-dress runners and ever-amusing quips from the crowds ('Can you turn me into a pumpkin?') provided all the distraction I needed. Someone I repeatedly encountered was Ladder Man, a runner carrying a six-foot-long ladder which he'd prop up against lamp posts and walls and clamber up and down before continuing running. I was going so slowly that even he kept overtaking me.

At the halfway mark on The Highway I spotted a beaming Uncle Ian brandishing balloons, a huge rainbow umbrella and a sackload of snacks. I don't think I've ever been happier to see someone I know. He informed me that Aunty Rosie was doing fine and was up ahead, and watched in amazement as I greedily scooped up half a dozen mini Mars bars, a bag of apricots, a handful of nuts and a pinch of raisins, and pressed on. The mile-long section along The Highway proved to be the most challenging of the entire course; it was a switchback where runners who'd run 13 miles shared the road with ones who'd already done 22. All that separated us was a flimsy bit of plastic tape. I spent the entire mile fighting the urge to duck under the tape and so take a nine-mile shortcut. 'No one will know,' said a little whiney voice in my head (most likely one of those Chinese crapping birds). 'Yes, but *I'll* know,' I had to keep repeating. And of course, as I now know, so too would the race officials, who would have been tipped off by my timing chip that I'd failed to cross several electronic timing mats.

What followed was the second-most challenging section of the course: the bit through the Isle of Dogs where, in those days, the crowd support was very sparse. By now my knee was so bad that I'd given up any pretence of running and was walking. I'd become accustomed to having my name called out at least every five seconds so to walk in silence – and in pain – proved very demoralising. Then something delightful happened: a woman came out of her house and offered me a sandwich. Although it was made from foamy white bread and 'plastic' ham it truly was one of the most delicious things I'd ever eaten. Having almost OD'd on sugary sports drinks, sweets, chocolate and dried fruit, eating something salty was utterly sublime. The sheer joy that a triangle of bread elicited almost made me cry. I wanted to find a wall to climb on so that I could make a speech about the goodness of humanity and the kindness of strangers. Of course I didn't do that – but now, looking back 16 years later, I wish I had.

I will always remember what happened at mile 20. At that precise point, somewhere on an almost-deserted highway in Poplar, I ran the step that meant I had just gone further than I'd ever gone in my entire life. Twenty miles! Thirty-two whole kilometres! I thought my heart was going to explode with pride. 'You're in new territory now,' I thought, 'you've never run this far, and you never will again, but you've done it!' Every cell, every muscle, every nerve in my body vibrated with this sense of success. I almost expected a marching band to materialise from the nearby petrol station to help me celebrate this magnificent milestone but, as the band obviously had better things to do, I tucked into a victory mini Mars bar instead. However, at 22.5 miles I had a major wobble. By now the blue line painted on the road to indicate the marathon route had been erased by a little van with sweeper brushes and I was in a tunnel, with no other runners in sight, unsure of whether I was still on track. Emerging from the gloom I found myself, in an almost comedic moment, on a red carpet. 'Huh?' I thought, momentarily suspecting I might be hallucinating from exhaustion. But then it dawned on me that I was on the notorious cobbled road next to the Tower of London and that the organisers had laid down the carpet to stop us from slipping – not to make us feel even more like A-listers. The final stretch along the Thames was where I'd spent so many evenings training. 'You've already run this bit – you own it, almost there,' I lied to myself as my feet began to protest just as loudly as my knees. This late in the day the course was full of families out for a Sunday stroll, and it became increasingly difficult to navigate my way through the crowds. Just then I was overjoyed when I spotted Karen, a South African schoolfriend I'd known since the age of 13, beaming at me on The Embankment. She'd witnessed my sport-hating ways on many occasions during my teenage years and, when she heard I was running the marathon, offered to come along both to support me and, I suspect, verify that I wasn't telling a whopper about participating!

After a couple of miles of chat-walking we heard someone shouting: 'Runner coming through!' and turned to see the race's oldest female participant, 87-year-old Jenny Wood-Allen, accompanied by two younger friends who were clearing her path. I'd read about Jenny in the pre-race publicity: when she first started marathon running aged 71, she'd felt so self-conscious as a woman with white hair and wrinkles that she'd taken a shopping bag along so that she could pretend she was just in a hurry to get to the shops. 'There's no way I'm letting a woman who's almost 90 beat me,' I thought grimly, trying to increase my pace. Just as Big Ben came into sight I watched in dismay as the tiny figure in a white fabric sunhat disappeared from view.

And then it happened: the moment I managed to salvage my battered pride. I saw Jenny again, and this time she'd stopped. Right outside the Houses of Parliament, where the course took a sharp right. Being a law-abiding pensioner she'd obeyed a red traffic light and was waiting for it to turn green. Spotting my chance I jaywalked across the junction and broke into an agonising shuffle. With just over half a mile to go I knew that if I walked so much as a single step Jenny would overtake me, so I dug as deep as I possibly could, put my head down and grimly hobbled down Birdcage Walk which, that day, was officially the longest, straightest, deadliest, dullest road in the known universe. Once again my mind was filled with fearful thoughts. I just didn't want to have to say I'd been overtaken by someone almost three times my age. I kept glancing backwards and each time I did so that brave little figure seemed to be gaining on me.

When I later looked up my results – 7h12 if you went by the clock or 6h55 if you went by my timing chip – I learned that I'd finished just over two minutes ahead of Jenny (whom I'd later have the honour of interviewing for *Running Made Easy*). Three years later, despite having sustained a head injury after a fall while training, Jenny bowed out of marathon running in style when she finished her last London Marathon in 11h34 at the grand old age of 90.

As I crossed under the yellow and green finish arch, tinsel-covered wand held high (and now only half full of jellybeans), I burst into floods of tears. It was the most horrendous and brilliant thing I'd ever done. Then one of the volunteers hung my medal round my neck and said: 'Well done, Lisa. You *really* deserve this.' I just couldn't get over the fact that this woman had probably been standing there for close to five hours, and hadn't just handed me my medal but had gone to the trouble of hanging it round my neck as if I was an Olympic champion, even taking the time to congratulate me by name. I wanted to give her a hug, but I knew that I'd only end up smearing tears, snot and sweat all over the poor woman, so I fought the urge and instead limped off to find my family. I had a joyful reunion with Alex and my aunt and uncle in St James's Park. Aunty Rosie had had an amazing time acting as an impromptu tour guide for a runner from South Africa, while Alex had run the entire race in panic mode and so, while achieving a good time, hadn't had a particularly fun one. When the hugging and medal stroking was over, I flopped heavily onto the grass and carefully removed my trainers. My feet were so painful that I genuinely expected blood to spurt from them as I did so. Truth be told, I was a bit disappointed when all I saw were a couple of blisters – there wasn't so much as a speck of blood on my socks.

'Never again!' I kept repeating to anyone who'd listen. 'I'm soooo pleased I've done it, but even more pleased that I *never* have to do it again.'

Much like new mothers forget what labour was like when gazing at their beloved newborn, a few days later, once the pain in my feet had abated somewhat, and despite my vows never to run another marathon, I was planning my next one. Looking back, I now realise this astonishing about-face was because I'd become addicted to the cheering. Hearing thousands of people chanting my name and willing me to succeed was the ultimate runner's high. The sense of achievement at having finished had almost entirely wiped out the memory of the agony involved in doing so. Despite Sally The Running Guru advising me that most runners only do one marathon a year, I decided to enter the Edinburgh Marathon that autumn as I was determined to actually run a marathon – not to walk half of it as my knee problem had forced me to do in London. I'd also decided that Edinburgh would be an opportunity for my husband to atone for an almost unpardonable sin he'd committed. Despite hearing constant reports on my training via email while he was in Bahrain, he'd failed to wish me luck for London and hadn't so much as asked how it had gone afterwards. A week of my failing to reply to his daily emails had finally prompted a phone call enquiring whether he'd done something wrong.

'Well, if you call ignoring the biggest achievement of my life "doing something wrong", then yes, you have,' I replied coldly.

'Oh no. I didn't!' he groaned. 'You haven't done London *already*, have you? I thought it was *next* week. I'm truly, *truly* sorry. Is there any way I can make it up to you?'

'Now that you mention it, there is. I want you to run the Edinburgh Marathon with me.'

'What? A whole marathon? Surely there must be another way I can apologise.'

'It's that or nothing,' I insisted. Five months later Graham and I were standing in a field in Dunfermline listening to a Scottish piper playing in the mist as we waited for the start gun. I'd loaded my bumbag with a huge hoard of snacks, including half a pound of dates, and had once again trained pretty hard. Graham, on the other hand, had barely run at all. I think his reasoning was that if I, the world's most fitness-averse specimen, could do a marathon, then pretty much anyone could.

'You really should train – even a little bit,' I'd urged him. So he reluctantly did a single 10K run that went so well he declared himself marathon-ready.

'Don't come crying to me if you struggle on the day,' I said.

'Never fear, I won't,' he replied smugly.

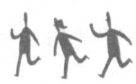

I'd vowed to run the whole way, without a single step of walking, even if it killed me. Which it almost did. I remember very little of the race except that Graham and I parted ways pretty much immediately as he hates talking while running – and I hate being with someone who stays silent even more. I was full of trepidation at the notion of trying to run nonstop, so I tried to distract myself from the scary 'what if I just can't' thoughts by hitching up with a chatty woman who'd admired my fairy outfit. We enjoyed marvelling at the views of the iconic Forth (Rail) Bridge as we ran across the adjacent Forth Road Bridge, but eventually I proved too slow and she went on ahead of me, leaving me to my own devices.

Keeping going was an enormous struggle. Somewhere midway through the race, while plodding along the coast near Leith, I began chanting 'I am fit, I am strong, I will run this marathon'. In the end I must have repeated this mantra several thousand times. Every part of me ached; my hips in particular hurt like hell. It was almost as if someone had yanked my legs out of their sockets, plunged them into a fire, and then pushed them back into my torso. With every step I groaned aloud. Even when I was joined by two elderly runners, I couldn't stop my guttural moaning.

'Don't worry, Fairy, we'll get you to the finish,' said the kindly grey-haired veteran of six marathons who was supporting his white-haired friend, who had a heavily bandaged knee, through his first marathon.

On we plodded, with me attempting to talk whenever I wasn't groaning. Along the way, when I realised I was running too hard to feel hungry, I reluctantly ditched the huge block of dried dates I'd brought along. Having dodged the throngs of Sunday shoppers and tourists in Princes Street we finally reached the finish line, where my surprisingly early arrival shocked a very weary, sore and chastened Graham. I had beaten my previous marathon time by a whopping 78 minutes, finishing *much* earlier than he'd anticipated. Having put on a huge fake grin for my official race photo, I dropped the pretence the minute I was no longer in front of the lens. Throwing myself down on the grass I burst out crying – and then realised Graham was photographing me.

'Take *lots* of photos of this,' I sobbed, 'because, if I'm ever crazy enough to be tempted to run another marathon I want a permanent reminder of how horrible this one was. I wouldn't wish this kind of pain on my worst enemy. I know I've said it before… but this time I really mean it: I am *NEVER* running a bloody marathon again.'

And Graham? Funnily enough he said pretty much the same thing (minus the tearful theatrics). The wheels had come off at mile 20 (32.2K) when he realised he just couldn't continue running. At that point he'd been joined by another runner and they'd both tried to cajole each other into running again, to no avail. It was a painful six miles (9.7K) to the finish, during which time not a single step was run, but he nonetheless posted a very respectable time of 4h36, exactly an hour faster than me. Graham soothed his battered ego by telling me that the other runner was a graduate of Sandhurst, the British Army's super-tough officer training centre. If a *soldier* from *Sandhurst* found Edinburgh tough, reasoned Graham, then the fact that he'd found it a bit of a challenge wasn't too shabby.

For three weeks after Edinburgh I had to walk down stairs backwards and the fire in my hips glowed undimmed. But it only took about a week before I started thinking about doing another marathon. 'I'd just like to get to five – that's a nice round number,' I told myself, 'and then I'll stop.' What I feared, however, was that if marathon running was going to take such a tremendous toll on my body I might end up in a wheelchair by the time I was 40. I really was terrified of crippling myself but knew that there was no point in denying it – I had definitely caught a really bad case of marathon fever.

Fear once again played a huge part in my third marathon. Paris is my favourite city so I was really looking forward to running there in the springtime to celebrate the new millennium. I'd done two months of training before it all skidded to a halt – one minute I was able to run 10K with relative ease, the next I could only get to 2K before agonising knee pain meant I couldn't go on. I continued to train on an elliptical trainer at the gym, determined to make a go of cramming in the miles come what may, but, just a fortnight before race day I found I still couldn't run more than a couple of kilometres. In a last-ditch attempt to salvage my race I consulted an osteopath who diagnosed a leg-length discrepancy and told me he was surprised that, with one leg so much shorter than the other, I didn't walk with a limp. He suggested I insert several heel lifts (small pieces of padded leather) into my left shoe, which I duly did, and miraculously the pain instantly disappeared.

The night before race day, however, I lay on my hotel bed, rigid as a plank with fear. Would the inserts be enough to get me through? 'You've got your stress face on,' observed my husband, trying to lighten the mood but only succeeding in focusing my mind on my anxiety. To help myself relax I started browsing through the race brochure and came across an article where an elite runner encouraged anyone who was unsure of their ability to finish to consider walk/running the race. I was desperate to try anything and so resolved to give it a go.

I felt horrendous the next day, partly because of fear but mostly because I hadn't slept at all. After a short Metro ride with my Aunty Rosie, who'd again offered to run with me, we set off in search of a loo, only to find that not one of the ten streets radiating out from the Arc de Triomphe seemed to have one. Growing desperate, my aunt marched me over to a small patch of lawn and, pulling me down into a crouching position, commanded: 'Wee! No one will see!'

And that's how I ended up peeing behind a few blades of grass on the Champs-Élysées with only a see-through tutu covering my modesty while thousands of runners ambled past on the way to the start line.

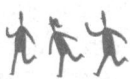

The Paris Marathon begins on a downhill slope so you have a dramatic view of the kaleidoscopic carpet that is 30,000 colourfully clad runners surging down the French capital's most prestigious avenue. Aunty Rosie had agreed to follow my new run/walk strategy by running for 15 minutes and then walking for five, but after 10K (6.2 miles) my knee suddenly twanged like an awkwardly plucked guitar string. Devastated, I slowed to a limp and told her to go on ahead. No sooner had she scooted off than the pain subsided and I was able to continue run/walking again. I found I really loved this new way of doing things: during the running segments I looked forward to having a walk break and, during the walk breaks, I rested and refuelled. What's more, my muscles didn't ache: it was almost like having two different sets of legs!

After running along the *quais* under the Seine's many bridges, where thousands of Parisians stood shouting encouragement, and shedding a tear while passing through the Pont de l'Alma tunnel where Princess Diana died, I emerged to see the Eiffel Tower beckoning me like a giant finger. I caught up with my aunt, who was walking with a veteran of 52 marathons, during the final stretch through the leafy Bois de Boulogne. When I urged them both to join me, my aunt told me there was no way she could contemplate running again and that I should borrow her companion and make a dash for it. Fearful that the 5h30 cut-off would be strictly applied (meaning I wouldn't get an official time or medal), I reluctantly set off with my aunt's French companion, whose infectious chatter spurred me on to run faster than I'd run all race. I actually sprinted the final 5K (3.1 miles), urged on by a troupe of transvestite pom-pom-waving cheerleaders, pausing only once to grab a plastic cup of wine offered to us by supporters in a wooded section of the park. When I crossed the finish line in 5h27 (an astonishing nine minutes faster than Edinburgh, where I'd run all the way) I broke into an enormous grin and once more vowed never to run a marathon again. But this time I meant it, because from now on, I decided, I would always be sure to walk/run.

So what has running taught me about fear? Overcoming my fear that April day in Paris in 2000 changed my life. When I lined up at the start, a huge part of me held on to the false expectation that I'd fail to finish, but when, instead of giving in to that fear as I would have done previously, I faced it head on, it eventually evaporated, and I reached the finish line fearless and triumphant. Never again would I let a fear of failure stop me from starting something.

That day in Paris also showed me that walking early on in a marathon could actually make you faster than running continuously. It was a relief to realise that walking wasn't a sign of weakness after all; it was a way of working smarter rather than harder. Best of all, it took me just three days to recover afterwards, a far cry from the three weeks it took me to walk normally again after the Edinburgh Marathon. I was so eager to share this newfound secret with other beginners, for whom running a marathon is often considered an almost impossible feat, that I resolved to write a book about it. But in order to do so I knew I'd have to overcome another major fear – the fear of being laughed at. Every running book I'd read up to that point was written by either a sports scientist, an elite runner or at least a gifted one, not someone like me who believes, as the saying goes, that 'life is short – and running makes it seem longer'. Who on earth was going to take running advice from someone at the very back of the marathon pack? So I shelved the idea, but a few months later realised that if I wanted to inspire other fitness-phobes like me to discover the joy of marathoning I had no option but to evict the squatters living rent-free in my head, the ones who appeared to be staging a dirty protest while chanting 'Who'd ever listen to you?', and force myself to start writing.

Facing down that second fear was life-changing, too. Together with my co-author Susie, a colleague at *Zest*, I realised that we didn't need to be experts to write about running: we just needed to quote the right experts! And when we contacted them we were humbled by the hugely generous way that runners such as Jeff Galloway (the legendary walk/run guru) and Professor Tim Noakes (a South African sports scientist acclaimed the world over) were prepared to share their knowledge. We soon found out that we were definitely not the only ones eager to spread the joyous word. Four years later my first book *Running Made Easy*, which expounded the walk/run concept, was published. It went on to sell over 100,000 copies and, in doing so, became Britain's best-selling beginners' running book. Since publication we've received countless emails from people thanking us for turning them into runners by 'legitimising' walk breaks. The book's success eventually led to my being appointed Contributing Editor at *Women's Running*, where I've given myself the title of The World's Slowest Marathon Correspondent and have had the privilege of travelling the world in search of remarkable races in spectacular places. I've also hosted running camps in the Alps, at which I've found that the biggest thing holding would-be runners back wasn't their ability (or supposed lack thereof), but the fear they felt of not being good enough to run faster or further.

Marathons are sometimes called 'Everyman's Everest' and every marathon I've done has given me the chance to do something I find difficult. The chance to conquer my fear – and *myself* – and to plant a flag in my mind, like successful summiteers do, that reads: 'Lisa runs. Who ever would've thought it?'

'We fought our fear – and won!'

'Running terrified me but I did it anyway'

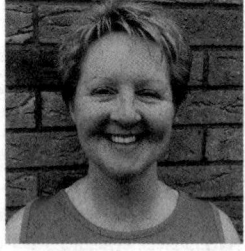

I'm actually a real scaredy cat. With every single thing I do I am frightened, without fail. And yet I haven't let this stop me going skydiving, paragliding, skiing, scuba-diving, firewalking – or taking up running. That's because I know if I allow myself to give in to fear, I'll never do anything exciting.

When I first started running my biggest fear was that I wouldn't be able to do it and that I'd look ridiculous, so I wore sunglasses and a baseball cap with a big peak pulled down. However, the main barrier was removed when I met a lot of lovely, like-minded people on Lisa's running camp in the Alps. I felt excited that I was finally running but mostly I felt heavy, sweaty, red-faced and breathless. Then I slowly began to realise that the only thing stopping me becoming a runner was 'me, myself and I', so when I got back home I started going to parkruns and joined a running group.

I ran my first 10K with Lisa and my fellow running-retreat guests in Bristol. We called ourselves Team No Fear and posing for a photo below the Clifton Suspension Bridge halfway round felt awesome. However, near the end I was totally panic-stricken as by then I was hobbling due to extreme knee and hip pain. I'd never run that far before and when Lisa told me no one ever walks the last kilometre of a 10K I'm sure my eyes came out on stalks like a cartoon character. I didn't want to let her or me down so I gritted my teeth – and did it! When the medal was hung round my neck I had to try hard not to bawl my eyes out, but they would've been happy tears, not sad ones. My motto? It has to be: 'Fight the fear and do it anyway!'

Dawn McLean, 56, Preston, Lancashire, England

'When I had depression, running threw me a lifejacket'

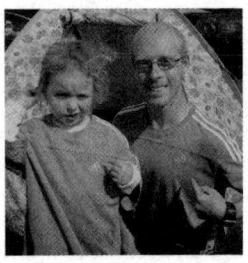

In 2010 my wife and I relocated to Wales and were expecting our first child. Moving away from home left me feeling isolated and I was overwhelmed by the pressures of my new job. Even though I knew I had supportive friends and family, I developed depression and feared I'd lose control of everything I held dear, including my own sanity. I became terrified of not being there to see my unborn daughter grow up. Fortunately my GP suggested cognitive behavioural therapy and exercise. I'd done a half marathon with my Dad three years before so I began running again and it helped me to focus my thoughts and showed me how lucky I am to have the life I do.

In 2012 I began training for the London Marathon. During one run my left knee gave out and I had to call my wife Anastasia to fetch me. I was distraught and thought it was all over but she gave me a good talking to and told me to take hot and cold baths and come back fighting the next day. I did as I was told and proceeded to give my legs the same stern talking to – and it worked. London was a fabulous experience and the next year I did another marathon. Then in July 2014 I set myself a 30 Marathons For 30 Years Challenge, which meant I had to run another 26 marathons before turning 30 in December 2015. I wanted to inspire my four-year-old daughter Issy, and everyone around me, and help them realise that if you want something badly enough you'll find a way to achieve it. When we asked Issy if she'd like to enter the Mini Great North Run she loved the idea and didn't need any convincing. Her main goal was 'to finish like Daddy' – and she did!

Martin Mead, 29, Essex, England

'A fear of embroidery drove me to run!'

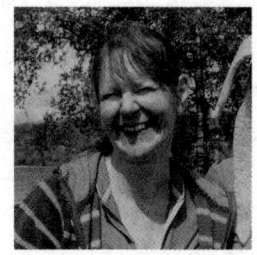

I guess you could say that fear has motivated me to run for the past seven years. Since turning 60 I've been scared of turning into the kind of woman who sits on her porch doing embroidery, so instead I've aspired to run 100 marathons.

The journey has certainly been an interesting one: since becoming a marathon runner aged 52 I've lost 5 stone (30 kg), achieved a marathon PB of 4h20 at the age of 63 and completed 46 marathons (21 of them in 2012 as a way to celebrate the Olympics coming to London). Popping down to the local pub to show off my first marathon medal also had unexpected consequences: I met the man I would later run off to Gretna Green with, my husband Allan.

An injury picked up in 2013 led to a fear that I'd never run marathons again. I couldn't finish three of the marathons I entered that year – and withdrew from 11 – so you can only imagine how much weeping went on. However, that's simply made me more determined to stick with my physio's rehab programme, which has made me realise the importance of strength and conditioning exercises that can help to prevent injury, such as the plank, press-ups and squats (I can now do longer squats than women a third of my age at the gym).

I met the legendary world's oldest marathon runner Fauja Singh once and he told me that one of the secrets of his success was avoiding negative people. I agree, and aim to avoid negative thinking, too. By facing my fears head on I've become the woman I am today – someone who's out running next to lakes and up hillsides, ponytail swinging. Someone who doesn't have time to do embroidery. I've learned to ignore the naysayers and run with my heart.

Penny Lovegrove, 67, Lake District, England

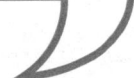

Before I ran, I was afraid. Afraid of looking like an idiot, yes, but also deep down scared to death that I wouldn't be able to do it. Years of me telling myself I couldn't do sport meant I set myself up to fail before I even ran one step. But I didn't fail. I ran. It was hard but not horrendous. So I ran some more. Before long, running was part of my weekly routine. I knew I had the running bug when I asked my hubby to buy me running shoes for Christmas instead of jewellery. But it wasn't just running I found I could do. I was trying new things: I jumped on trampolines, climbed trees, splashed about in the pool with my four kids. I felt fit and alive. I had fun again!

Kelly Owen, 38, Cheltenham, England

I thought running would be like *über*-walking when I started. It's much worse. My legs felt unbelievably heavy and I thought I might cough up a lung. Ever run away from an axe murderer in a dream but you can't scream and your legs don't work? Like that. I started running for a minute at a time with walking breaks, and worked up to running for 20 minutes solidly. I was amazed at how quickly it got easier. Apparently my body got stronger... I think of it as being able to escape the axe murderer a little more quickly. I still have the brief 'axe-murderer five minutes' at the start of each run, but it's soon over and I can't say I've ever been sorry I went out.

Iona Bower, 36, Horsham, England

I've had a flying phobia for 16 years and last year, having recently started running, got the chance to enter the 261 Women's 10K. The only problem was that I had no option but to fly there as it takes place on the island of Majorca. Running had started to make me feel strong and taught me that the only thing limiting me was myself, so I dared myself to do it. When I boarded the plane I felt equally excited and frightened but when we landed I felt the same sensation one does when crossing the finish line: immensely empowered. The race was amazing, too – I met many wonderful women and it felt as if we were all sisters.

Marga Gómez, 43, Madrid, Spain

A collision with a drunk driver in 2000 left me with a bent spine (and a useless sports-science degree) so my initial fear was that I'd never run again. Intensive physiotherapy helped me overcome that fear and in 2012 I decided to run my first marathon. The buzz on getting my medal was so intense that I ran quite a few marathons that year, culminating in doing 58 for charity in 2014. I have to rely on painkillers to get me through, especially when I'm running several marathons in a week, but I never let my fear of not finishing stop me from starting.

Vicky Horne, 35, Hampshire, England

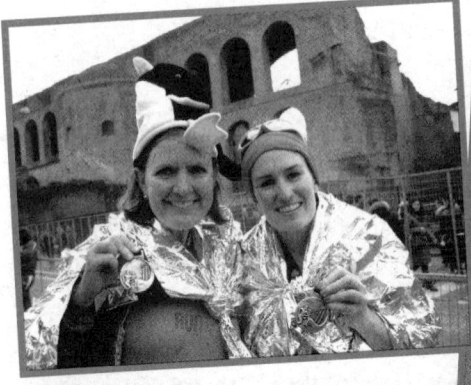
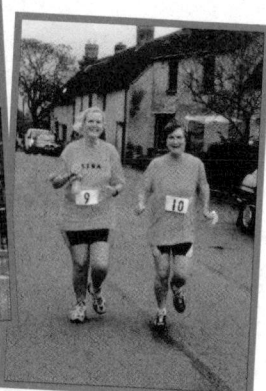
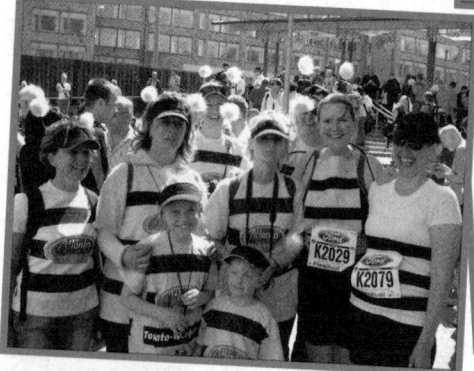
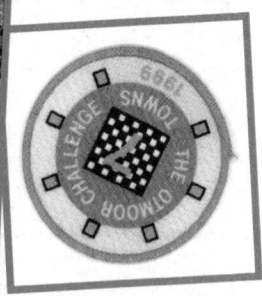
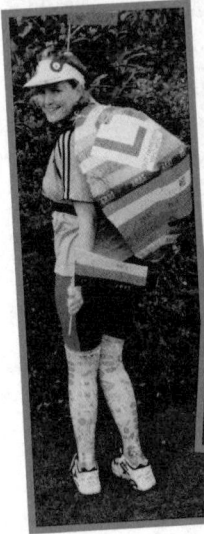
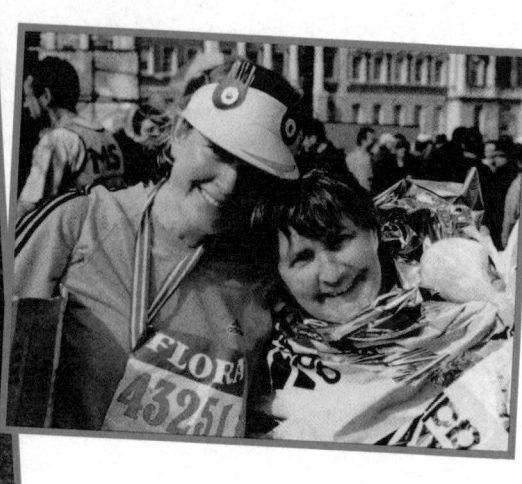

Chapter 3

What running taught me about... never, never, never giving up

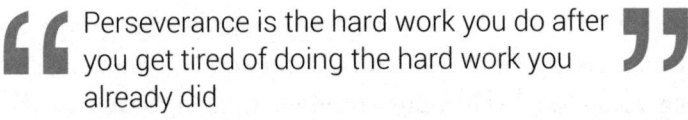 Perseverance is the hard work you do after you get tired of doing the hard work you already did

Newt Gingrich

If there's one thing in life that distance running teaches you in spades it's digging deep. Whether you're hobbling or hotfooting it round a half, full or ultramarathon, the lactic acid in your limbs will inevitably, at one point or another, find its voice and start shouting for you to stop the insane activity you're engaged in and have a nice little sit-down. In fact, you're lucky if it's only the lactic acid talking. There's a little spiteful-faced monkey who lives inside my head and he's got a pain threshold a helluva lot lower than my legs have. Whereas I usually find that it's just beyond the halfway point of any race that the lactic acid starts whining away, the evil monkey (I like to think of him with wings, just like those terrifying flying monkeys in the *Wizard of Oz*) jumps in much sooner, and because those wings make him more mobile, you never quite know when he's going to start mouthing off. My monkey is a world champion sofa-surfer with Olympic medals in any activity that involves sitting or lying down. He does not like sport, activity or exercise because they make him, well, tired. During every event I've entered my monkey has put up a protest as early as he possibly can.

Take the Otmoor Challenge, for example. I entered this half marathon in the curiously named Horton-cum-Studley in Oxfordshire two months after my first marathon at the insistence of my Aunty Rosie, who lived nearby. It all started amicably enough. The start was slap bang in the middle of a village fete that advertised quaint country activities such as sheep racing, and the route promised stunning views of the Seven Towns of Otmoor, a conservation area renowned among twitchers for its abundant birdlife.

We set off at an average chat-run pace of 10,000 words a minute, revelling in the tourist-brochure-pretty countryside, without the faintest idea of the horrors to come. 'Ah, life is good when you're a runner,' I thought as the other participants faded from view. Just then the course became a bridleway. How delightfully 'country', you might think. It wasn't. Ever heard the playground joke: 'What's brown and sticky?' The answer's supposed to be 'A stick.' But in this case it wasn't. The answer in this instance was 'Mud'. Whole skiploads of it. What had once been a track had been transformed into a mudbath by the preceding day's torrential rain. What's worse, it ponged of horse poo. Wherever the horses had gone past their hooves had somehow created little molehill-sized mounds, so whenever I put my foot down it would land on top of one and then slide right off it, like chocolate sauce being poured onto a ball of ice cream.

The monkey landed on my shoulder with a bone-shaking screech seconds later. 'Stop!' it commanded. 'You're going to break your ankle. I cannot allow this insanity to continue for a moment longer!' For a minute or so I seriously considered quitting, but I didn't have a clue where we were so I had no choice but to tell my monkey to put a sock in it and continue to gingerly pick my way along the mounds at a pace of just ten words a minute, most of which were curses. At long last I made it to the end of the bridleway and looked down at my trainers, which felt as if they'd been filled with concrete. I was amazed to see that, snowball-like, they'd collected layers of mud with each step and now resembled the oversized feet of Minnie Mouse. With my monkey doing a stomping Rumpelstiltskin impression on my shoulder to show his displeasure at being both silenced and ignored, I lurched over to a fencepost and began kicking it (the post, not the monkey). Bit by bit huge chunks of caked-on mud fell off like icebergs shearing off a glacier. By now it had started to rain, which made navigation even more difficult, but we decided to soldier on.

It was after we'd been sloshing along a farm track for an hour that we saw them, dimly through the drizzle. There must have been at least 30 of them, and they were all looking straight at us. It's a little-known fact that there are 11 animals more likely to kill you than sharks, and cows – which look deceptively placid – are one of them. I'm a city girl through and through and 'Trampled by Killer Cows' was not what I wanted to have engraved on my gravestone, so I clutched my aunt's hand and urgently whispered that we should retreat before they stampeded over to get a closer look.

'Nonsense,' said Aunty Rosie, 'we're going through!'

And so, fixing the cows with our most intense stares we hastily traversed the field only to find, on exiting it, that we were lost. And as there were no other runners in sight to lead the way, we had no choice but to retrace our steps, hearts racing even though our feet no longer were. (Sixteen years later, during the Weald Challenge Trail Marathon, I would learn that a better way to deal with curious cows is to shout 'Moooove away! Moooove away!' – no pun intended – in your most authoritarian voice and run right at them, rather than try to skulk past them.) We managed to find the arrows indicating the route again, just in time to face our next challenge: the course's most horrendous hill. Just then my Uncle Ian, who'd once again come along to support us, pulled up in his car. Boy, were we glad to see him – but our joy only lasted a few seconds because his encouragement consisted of the dispiriting words: 'Get a move on, the marshals want to go home!'

When we finally made it back to the fete, my uncle came rushing over with a huge umbrella in one hand and two cups of tea clutched precariously in the other.

'Get under this,' he urged.

'Get away from us,' hissed Aunty Rosie. My poor uncle looked very taken aback.

'We haven't crossed the finish line yet!' she cried.

As we frantically scanned the field trying to locate it, the race director scurried over: 'You took so long to arrive we've taken the finish line down,' he grinned while presenting each of us with a small fabric cub-scout-like badge, 'but you deserve these more than most!' Never had tea tasted so good. Never had a tracksuit badge been viewed as a badge of courage. And never had the words 'Never again' been uttered with more conviction (and this time I really did mean it – I've *never* been back!).

My running career is littered with examples of the times my perseverance – or, as my husband would deem it, my 'stubbornness' – has been my secret ninja skill. For example, my second London Marathon in 2001, which I ran in box-fresh new shoes. Of course *Runner's World* had told me not to, but I didn't have any other option. As my osteopath had suggested, I had been using heel lifts in my left shoe to balance out my leg-length discrepancy. The only problem was, I needed about six of the darn things, and using so many pushed my left heel up and out of my shoe, meaning there was no support for my ankle. It was like running on a pile of wobbly Scotch pancakes.

Having run with my heel lifts for nine months, I visited a running shop to buy a new pair of trainers. When the shop assistant spotted my home-made leg extension she said she was astounded that it hadn't resulted in a twisted ankle and suggested I visit a local shoemaker who'd be able to strip out some of the cushioning in my right shoe. This would allow my legs to be the same length and hence I wouldn't need to use the heel lifts. When I fetched my trainer from the shop the thought did cross my mind that he had in fact stripped *all* of the cushioning out. However, as the shoemaker had been recommended to me by a running expert, I didn't think to question this further and continued with my training which, among other things, involved running three half-marathon distances. In the same way that your hand would be bruised if you slammed it into your kitchen table wrapped only in a tea towel for protection, my right foot was so badly battered come marathon day that I could hardly walk. I rushed out to buy yet another pair of new trainers and hence lined up at the start line wearing ones so virginal I could've drunk champagne out of them. I soon found out why this is often cited as Marathon Crime #1. You know how satisfying it is to play with bubble wrap? Well, it's not when the bubble wrap is your feet – and each bubble represents a plasma-packed blister. I know for a fact that I would never have managed to hobble all the way from Blackheath to Buckingham Palace if I hadn't had Aunty Rosie by my side, and if I hadn't put my ninja stubbornness skill to good use with every agonising step.

My aching feet made another cameo appearance in the 2013 Rome Marathon. Race day coincided with the newly elected Pope Francis's first blessing in St Peter's Square, meaning the Eternal City would be packed with 200,000 pilgrims as well as 11,000 runners. This proved a major headache for the organisers, who had to come up with a new route to enable the race to go ahead.

With the Colosseum as an epic backdrop, I could sense that many of us were having a Spartacus moment as we got ready to set off. This feeling wouldn't last. The previous time I'd run the Rome Marathon in 2004 there had been, at most, 2K (1.2 miles) of cobbles, or *sampietrini* as they're known there. This time there must've been 20K (12.4 miles). Stone *is a lot* less forgiving than tarmac. Imagine grabbing hold of a hammer and spending over three hours striking the soles of your feet with it. Exactly. Neither the half dozen military bands playing stirring marching music nor the 500 historic sights such as the Circus Maximus and Trevi Fountain that we passed en route made a blind bit of difference to the pain I was in. Even seeing three guilty-looking nuns heading to St Peter's Square by squeezing past the crowd-control barriers and then sneaking across the course like naughty schoolgirls wasn't enough to distract me from my battered feet. It was only when I met another British runner doing her first marathon who was far worse off than I was that things started looking up. This runner had shattered her elbow in a cycling accident three months previously, which required an operation to repair it, and had then fallen off her bike again just three weeks before the race. What got me round was swapping running yarns interspersed with cobble-cursing while trying to find her a good place to pee (in the end I chose a gap between two trucks, realising too late that one of them had the driver inside). By the time we finally claimed our medals we'd resumed feeling like the all-conquering Roman gladiators we undoubtedly were, but it was only our sheer obstinacy that got us to the finish line.

Many, many times throughout my running life I've had to reach down into my soul to fish for courage that I wasn't sure was there, and every time I've been surprised at the sheer resilience and emotional strength we humans can muster when we need to. I'll mention only one more example: the 2006 Stockholm Marathon, which was held on one of the hottest days of the year. I'd entered this race with Bridget, a South African schoolfriend now living in Canada whom I'd recently got back in touch with after discovering she too was a runner, and her husband Kent. Bridget had run the Paris Marathon with me the year before and had roped Kent into doing his first marathon with us in the Swedish capital. The heat was truly unbearable and all three of us were so worried about not finishing that I conducted an impromptu hypnosis session as we lay on the lawn of the sports stadium in the blazing sunshine waiting for the 2pm start. When we finally got going it felt like running over a million hairdryers all set on max: the tarred road surface seemed to absorb the heat and then blast it back up, twice as hot. Even the bikini-clad samba dancers cheering us on in front of the Royal Palace looked overdressed in temperatures that must have reached 35°C. Never have more cups of water gone over me instead of into me as I struggled to keep going. When I reached into my bumbag for my customary chocolate bar at the 30K (18.6-mile) mark it had liquefied and squirted all over my arm like a volcano. The final few kilometres really took it out of me – I was trying to avoid catching sight of a man wearing a full bear suit as I'd been convinced he was going to get heatstroke ever since noticing his tomato-red face during the first kilometre. I just didn't want to be the last face he saw before he died. (Fear not, the shaggy bear lived, and I shared a hairy hug with him at the finish.) I was frantically trying to work out our race splits as I wasn't sure if Bridget and I would beat the six-hour cut-off, having spent a lot of the first half of the race running backwards shouting encouragement to Kent, who'd reluctantly dropped out around the halfway point due to injury. At one point we passed an aid station where they were handing out dextrose energy tablets, which taste like sugary antacid medication. 'Don't take any of those,' I warned Bridget, shuddering and wrinkling my nose at the memory of the last time I'd been given one mid-race by my aunt. 'They're utterly disgusting and will make you feel sick.' Bridget took one regardless. 'At this point, if I had to eat cockroaches to get me to the finish I would,' she said, cheerily crunching the chalky pellet. From that day onwards, 'eating cockroaches' became yet another code for perseverance. And it worked. Being cooled down by bystanders brandishing water pistols (and laughing with Bridget about eating cockroaches) gave us just enough energy to drag ourselves to the finish. The sight of Stockholm's wonderfully old-fashioned, red-brick 1912 Olympic Stadium, where 83 world records have been broken, was one of my happiest race moments yet – as was seeing the relief on my husband's face that we'd finished just in time to get a medal. 'I dreaded what you'd be like if, after all that, you'd come away empty-handed,' he said later. 'You would've been *hell* to go home with!'

My favourite tale of perseverance isn't my own, however. It's that of a group I ran with at the 2004 New York City Marathon. It was while researching case studies for *Running Made Easy* that I encountered Achilles International, an organisation set up in the States to encourage disabled people to participate in mainstream athletics. After interviewing Dikeledi Mosiane, a South African runner who'd had one of her legs amputated at the knee but had nonetheless run three marathons on crutches, I was invited to be one of her three guides. Guiding is hard work – Dikeledi pushed down on my arm with every stride, so it was like doing thousands of bicep curls non-stop. But whatever we guides went through was nothing compared with what Dikeledi endured. Within a mile of the start her new prosthetic leg started playing up and we had to stop, remove it, apply blister plasters and baby powder, and reattach the leg. This was a process we repeated virtually every mile. Dikeledi pressed on, never complaining, never tiring of all the terrible jokes and boring running stories we told her to keep her spirits up. At one point we passed someone even more physically challenged than she was: a man in a wheelchair who had no strength in his arms and who could only kick feebly at the ground to propel himself forwards. He had several guides accompanying him, but he never once let them push him – he was determined to complete the full distance under his own steam. Dikeledi revelled in the crowd support and marvelled at the skyscrapers and the apartment buildings festooned with encouraging banners residents had put up. Finally, after nine hours and 59 minutes, we crossed the finish line, and I promptly burst out crying. Dikeledi had no time for tears: she just beamed from ear to ear as her medal was hung around her neck. And a few minutes later our hero in a wheelchair arrived to a winner's welcome, toeing himself over the line, without help, as he'd vowed he would. Back at our hotel we heard many stories of what perseverance meant to those in our group. One Achilles runner, Marc, had, apparently, found the marathon so tough that at one point he'd said: 'Leave me, just leave me, leave me at the side of the road to die.' Another guide accompanying a blind runner had slipped on paper cups at a refreshment station. Not wanting to let her buddy down, she'd continued to the finish, from where she'd been rushed to hospital. The diagnosis? A broken ankle. She'd run half a marathon on it. And me? I found that marathon one of my toughest yet: ten hours on your feet doing bicep curls is extraordinarily taxing. When I finally got to bed that night I found a blister the size of a fried egg on one of my feet. But if I'd found it hard, I can only imagine what Dikeledi must have gone through that day.

So what has running taught me about perseverance? Almost everything I know about it, actually. Grinding out the miles when it has long since ceased to be fun has trained me to plug away and complete things even after the novelty's worn off, which proved invaluable when it came to setting up my hypnotherapy practice. And also when it came to writing books. Any would-be writer will tell you of the irresistible appeal of ironing your underwear the moment you're faced with a blank page – even Robert Louis Stevenson apparently didn't enjoy writing all that much; what he did like, however, was 'having written'. Running's taught me to keep my eyes lifted upwards and focused on the end result rather than allowing them to drift downwards to see all the hurdles and the often tedious hard graft that stand in the way. It's taught me to tell my inner monkey to shut up *and* ship out. It's also taught me that, just like Mr Humphrys says on *Mastermind*, if you've started, you might as well finish. It's taught that stubbornness is a virtue, not a vice. And that all running involves pain. There's the pain of discipline and there's the pain of regret. Sticking with the discipline is most definitely the well-paved path to success. By failing to stick with it, and heeding that wicked winged monkey, you'll experience something far more painful than the pain of pushing on – the pain of regret. And we all know that *that* kind lasts a lifetime.

'We will prevail'

'Cancer won't stop me running 100 marathons'

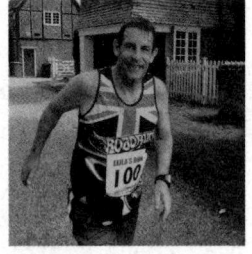

I was diagnosed with aggressive prostate cancer nine months ago and was told it had spread, so I had an operation to remove 13 lymph nodes, three of which were cancerous. I had 18 weeks off work due to the surgery, but then I got back on the road and started running marathons again as it's my goal to join the 100 Marathon Club. I'm a lorry driver and I started running at the age of 47 because I wanted to keep the weight off – most of my colleagues are obese. I've now run 115 half marathons and 91 marathons all over the world.

It's been hard physically and emotionally since getting the big C. I used to be a four-hour marathoner but now I struggle to finish before the cut-off times. One of the toughest races I've ever run was the Stroud Trail Marathon: it took me 10h48 and they kept the course open specially for me. The hilly route involved clambering over 30 stiles – and rock climbing in places – but I was determined to finish. I believe I'm able to persevere through the pain, come what may, for one reason: passion. Marathoning is something I really love. I'm now facing seven weeks of gruelling radiotherapy but no one has told me to stop running, so I won't.

I still have a lot to live for and have two main goals: to wear my 100 Marathon Club vest while doing the Walt Disney World Dopey Challenge in Florida (a 5K, 10K, half and full marathon all in one long weekend) and to wear it during my ninth London Marathon next year. I've told my seven-year-old granddaughter Eloise that I'm going to give her the medal all 100 Marathon Club members receive on completing their hundredth. She keeps reminding me of my promise, and I'll never let her down.

Steve Eaton, 60, Tamworth, Staffordshire, England

On 16 August 2015 I was honoured to be present when Steve Eaton achieved his dream of joining the 100 Marathon Club.

'Running the Amsterdam Marathon was like slogging through melted cheese'

I entered the Amsterdam Marathon because my friend Leroy said it would be a good idea. He'd completed a few marathons over the years and raved about the experience. And so I found myself trudging along a never-ending canal while a super-chirpy Leroy trotted beside me. I say chirpy but 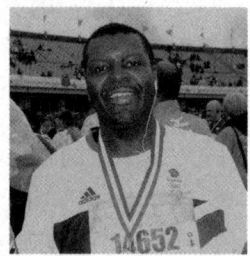 I didn't realise immediately that he was in fact suffering underneath too. Everyone seemed to be having a good time – except me.

At the canal section we got a wake-up call from the motorcycle outrider accompanying the dreaded sweeper van. He warned us that we weren't going to make the six-hour time limit which was a real kick in the backside and teeth at the same time. Leroy suggested we run between two lamp posts and then walk between the next two, which gave us achievable mini targets. My left ankle was killing me,

I was limping and I felt as if I was slogging through melted cheese. At several points we encountered Lisa — she was hard to miss in her cow hat — and she kept reminding me that I had to savour every second as I'd never be a marathon virgin again. Bloody right I wouldn't. I was never, never *ever* going to run another marathon. I again urged Leroy to run ahead and get his medal as I didn't want him to miss getting one because of me and he reluctantly left me, giving me some respite from the pressure of holding him back.

Towards the end there was a young woman wandering along, totally disoriented, picking up burst balloons and trying to eat them. It was odd to see how we humans can push ourselves so far beyond our natural limits that we're no longer capable of thinking rationally. When I finally reached the Olympic Stadium I was in shock at actually finishing. But the minute they hung that medal round my neck all the exhaustion, punishment, blisters, aches and many pains were worth it!

Roland, 48, London, England

'I've run almost daily for 60 years'

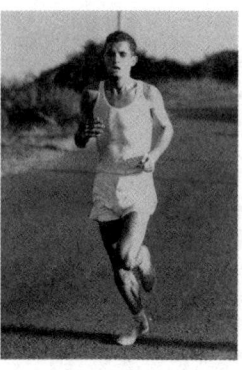

At high school I enthusiastically took part in sports day, but as a skinny 13-year-old I didn't win any races as I was competing against faster and older boys. Aged 16 I started training for longer distances and my housemaster allowed me to go out all alone after prep on 5K training runs through the pitch-black streets of Bloemfontein in South Africa. I wasn't scared in the least and simply relished the feeling of freedom. The result was that I won the school cross-country, and did so again the following year. At the age of 18 something utterly, utterly surprising happened: I won the half-mile and mile events against top athletes from the entire province in the Orange Free State Junior Championships.

When I was at university I continued running, and would never miss a training session, even if it meant going out late at night after a dance! Then in 1958, again unexpectedly, I won the South African University Cross-Country Championship, beating Jon Lang who went on to become a Springbok [international] marathon runner. I came second to Jon the following year, and these performances led me to think that I possibly had an international athletic career ahead of me. However, I soon realised that although I had the commitment, I lacked the required special genes, so I focused on getting my engineering degree instead. After university, I continued running almost daily and it became a way of life. Every day I'd get home from work and head out for a 5K or 6K run. At one point I was on the management board of an organisation with 5,000 employees and I found running an invaluable way to de-stress and clear my head. Over many decades I ran one half marathon a year and also completed two 50K ultramarathons.

I encouraged all three of my children to run – in fact, they say I nagged them into going running but I don't recall doing that. I just reasoned that what's good for me would be good for them, too. I love running, it's as simple as that, and wanted my kids to share the feeling. I was delighted when both of my daughters tackled the 91K Comrades Marathon. My proudest moment was when my youngest daughter Loren, who'd just finished a law degree, ran the Comrades having barely done any training. She was intending to drop out along the course but persevered and, having been awarded her medal, ended up in hospital with hyponatremia [low blood sodium levels due to drinking too much water, which can be fatal if untreated]. I was astounded when Lisa, who's not a fast runner, and hadn't run for years, ran her first marathon. Truth to tell, I was a bit concerned that she'd overdo it. But I'm very proud that she kept setting targets: her goal of doing 100 marathons is, frankly, unbelievable!

Now, 60 years after starting, I still run 6K every day. Running makes me feel good: if I don't go for a run for a day or two I feel uncomfortable and can't wait to get back to it. Now that I'm retired, I run to the gym every day, do some weights, then pop into my favourite pub for an ice-cold draft beer, and then run 3K home again. If anyone asks me how to keep a lifelong running routine going, I suggest a similar reward system!

Anthony Jackson, 76, Pretoria, South Africa

'I was seen as a weirdo
sweating my way to the finish'

I decided to run the Istanbul Marathon because it offers the unique opportunity to run a marathon on two continents. I instantly fell in love with the city – it's so exotic with its *Arabian Nights* mosques and gorgeous bay area. Five months before the marathon, political demonstrations had been held in 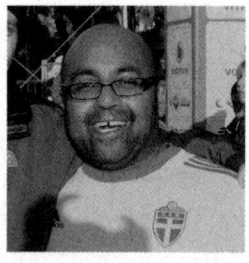 Taksim Square and there had been teargas and rubber bullets flying everywhere. I considered pulling out but my wife quipped: 'All the more reason for you to train harder so you can run away faster.'

I hadn't done enough training, so by the time I met Lisa 22K (13.7 miles) into the race my legs were seizing up and I was considering quitting. My mind was shouting at me to keep going – but my body was screaming 'No!' right back at it. Since I was in no fit state to engage in any normal conversation I didn't mind Lisa offloading all her troubles onto me (which she's since assured me she'd never done before or since): her luggage had been delayed at the airport so she'd almost missed collecting her race number at the Expo, and she'd be lucky to get a medal at all as we were in danger of missing the 5h30 cut-off time. Those few kilometres of chatting allowed my body to recover and so when we reached 28K (17.4 miles) I bid Lisa good luck and sprinted off. But soon my body started to seize up again. This was when I felt the loneliest as a runner. Earlier in the day I was cheered on but now, as one of the very few runners left on the course, I was seen as some weirdo, sweating and spluttering his way to the finish through the Sunday-afternoon shoppers. After crossing the finish line the intense pain and mental anguish gave way to euphoria. I couldn't believe I'd done it – I'd actually managed to run from Asia to Europe on my own two aching feet.

Rajnish Singh, 44, Brussels, Belgium

'I don't let temperatures of minus 30°C stop me from running outdoors'

I grew up in South Africa, where it snows once every 20 years, so moving to Winnipeg, one of the coldest cities in the world, took some getting used to. Lisa, whom I went to high school with (and with whom I now run a marathon at least once a year), thinks I'm utterly crazy 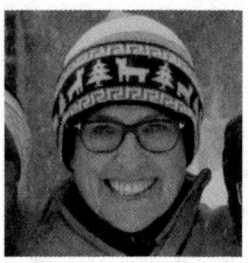 for running in extreme temperatures that'll frost your eyelashes in the blink of an eye. However, it's entirely doable provided you take certain precautions such as waiting until it warms up a bit when it's colder than minus 40°C. I use a spreadsheet to track what to wear for different temperatures and wind chills. The key is to wear layers, including a fitted Merino base layer. I'm also very careful with what I wear on my head. When I first started running in winter I asked my husband Kent, who's lived in Winnipeg all his life, if it was cold enough for a beanie, and he said no. When I got home and had a hot shower I screamed in pain. My ears were fat, red and stiff. Kent then informed me that they would, in all probability, turn black and fall off! Mercifully he was only teasing and they eventually got better and peeled, as if sunburnt. Now I always wear a hat and, if there's a wind chill warning, a neoprene facemask with a hood over the nose and mouth holes. I also cover any exposed skin on my face in Vaseline. Other than that, I just wear my summer shoes with wool socks.

There's a real sense of accomplishment at the end of a winter run and a heightened appreciation for a warm room and a hot drink. Running in extreme conditions has both an absurdity and levity to it — it makes you feel both adventurous and invincible.

Bridget Robinson, 47, Winnipeg, Canada

Seven marathons in seven days. The challenge isn't to finish each day, it's to start the next. All you want to do is go back to sleep, but you groan, grit your teeth and get up. Not because you have to – no one *has* to do this. You get up because you've set yourself a challenge. And not completing the challenge would mean you're letting yourself down. You could look everyone else in the eye. But you couldn't look yourself in the mirror with your head held high. So you force yourself to get up, feeling like you're 100 years old. And look in the mirror and tell yourself you're going to do it; you're going to start; and you're going to finish.

James Pattison, 41, County Durham, England

Leading the four-hour pacing group in the Milton Keynes Marathon was a huge responsibility as I had to become a human metronome and consistently run 9.09-minute miles. So how does one encourage a bunch of runners you've never met before to persevere no matter what? One of my secret weapons was to play music out loud and get my group singing along to old-time classics like The Jackson Five's 'ABC'. I also encouraged them to yell out 'Thank you, marshal!' every time we passed a volunteer. But most importantly I shouted out 'Showboat time, guys!' whenever we got within range of a photographer, so all my runners had time to put on their best race face.

Sunny Calitz-Patel, 48, London, England

'Running helped me feel normal after a brain tumour operation'

In 2008 I had an emergency operation to remove a brain tumour that left me with permanent double vision — it's like being drunk without the alcohol. When I left hospital my world had changed. I was unable to drive and I could no longer participate in the activities I'd previously enjoyed.

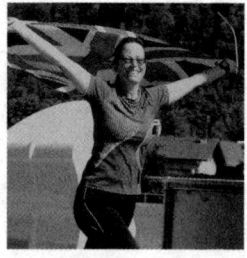

I certainly didn't plan on becoming a runner. One freezing winter's morning I missed the bus to work and, as it was too cold to stand and wait for another one, I started walking to the next stop just over a kilometre away. Then I realised that this was a bad mistake because the bus would probably pass me on the way, so I started running. I ran to the next bus stop, got there before the bus arrived, and felt exhilarated and so alive. Also, I was doing something that 'normal' people did. Until that point my visual impairment had been a tremendous handicap and I'd suffered severe bouts of depression. I felt incomplete as a person. But here was something I could do on equal terms with others. I was reborn and there was no stopping me, even though I found it hard to judge steps and kerbs and had to be very careful when crossing roads as when I turn my head everything is a jumble and I have to concentrate really hard until it makes any sense. The bug had bitten and I wanted to do more, so I completed the NHS Couch to 5K programme and started exploring local routes where I could run. That first year I entered the 10K Naisten Kymppi, a women-only event in Helsinki, and discovered how much fun it was to run in a race. The following year I signed up for a running course in the Alps led by Lisa and the year after that I did my first marathon with the friends I'd made there. Running has certainly pushed me out of my comfort zone, and it's taught me that perseverance brings its own rewards.

Fran Danilewicz, 56, Finland

'I simply refused to believe my marathon days were over'

Since I started in 1995 running has always been hugely important to me: I was the Launch Editor of *Women's Running* and a veteran of dozens of races. Then, while training for my second marathon, I felt a weird snapping sensation in my left knee, which swelled up like a balloon. I consulted 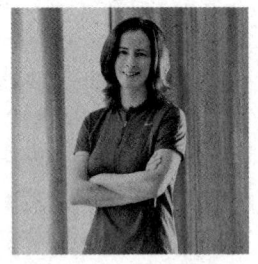 a renowned knee surgeon and, after having an MRI scan, went to see him for the results. Before I'd even had the chance to take my coat off, he said: 'The medial meniscus [cartilage] in your knee is torn and I can't fix it. Your marathon days are over. You won't run again.' I left his office in a daze and almost burst into tears.

After an operation to trim the torn parts of the meniscus to stop it further irritating my knee joint, I had lunch with Lisa, one of my contributors. She encouraged me not to give up, so I consulted my physio and began the long process of strengthening the muscles around my knee to give it as much protection as possible. Six months later I ran/walked my first 5K and the following year I ran four half marathons.

I never thought I'd run a second marathon even though I'd always wanted to do the London Marathon, but my physio said if I was sensible in training and did plenty of gym work I could give it a go.

The sense of community spirit on marathon day was amazing, with complete strangers offering me sweets, cakes, bananas and water. I found the last ten miles challenging but I didn't experience any knee pain. Running London made me realise that, if you really want to do something and someone says you can't, you shouldn't be afraid to challenge their opinion. My solution was really quite simple: positive thinking, strength work and controlling the frequency of my runs. It was a strategy that enabled me to fulfil a lifelong dream.

Chris Macdonald, 47, London, England

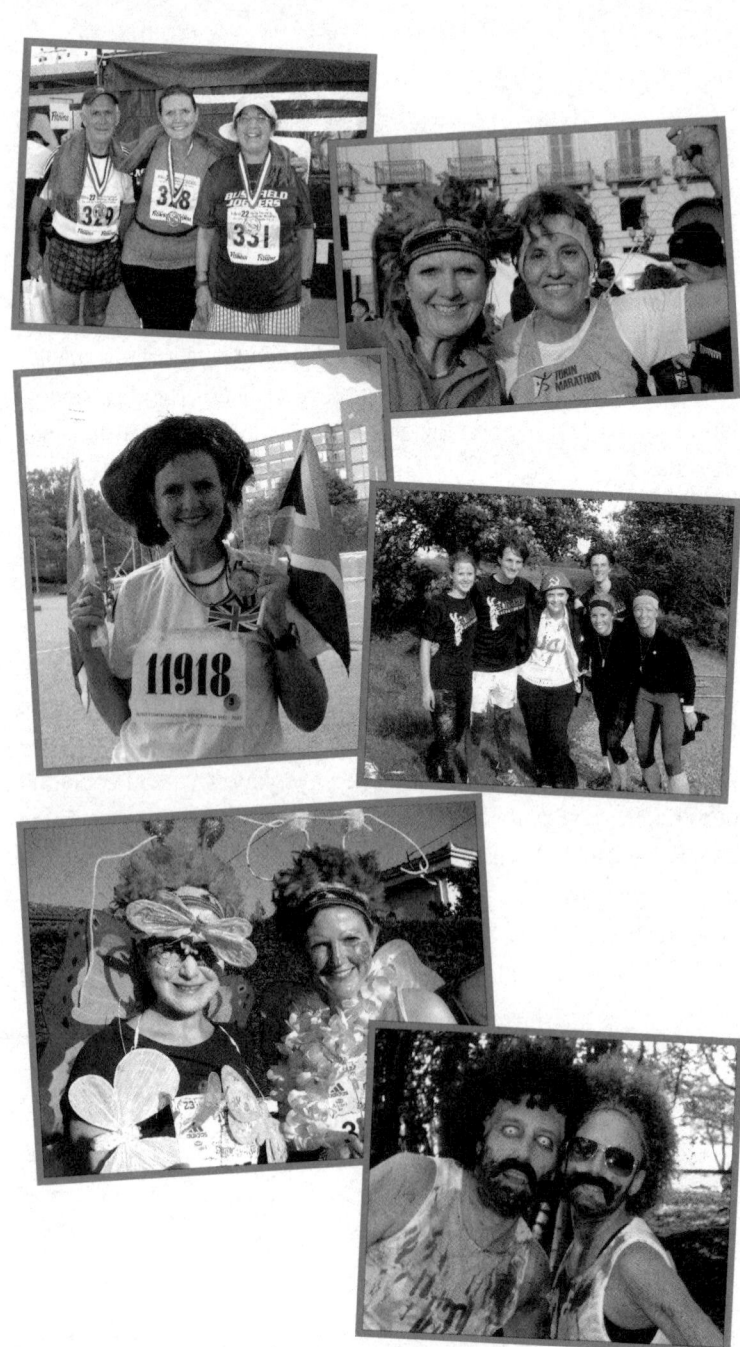

Chapter 4

What running taught me about... laughing

Running is good for your bones. Pavement pounding sends cells called osteoblasts to the bone surface to strengthen it. But there's one bone that it benefits above all others: the funny bone. I can't think of anything else I've ever done in life that's made me laugh as long and as hard as running has.

So where exactly have I found these mirth-making moments? Usually in the most unexpected places: a semi-deserted beach in France, for example. It was early on in my marathon career and I was, at that point, open to any ideas that would make me faster – even ones that sounded more dubious than a spam email promising me $15 million if only I'd pretend to be the next of kin of a deceased dictator. My sister had told me that I needed to learn to pee on the run – and no, she didn't mean stopping midway through a race, but actually *while* running. She informed me that many legendary South African ultrarunners use this technique and that it wasn't as disgusting as it sounds.

'You simply wee and then splash yourself with water afterwards, as if you're trying to cool yourself down,' she informed me. 'No one will be any the wiser.'

My chance to try this technique presented itself during a weekend camping trip to Wissant, France, which boasts a ten-kilometre-long sandy beach with views of the white cliffs of Dover across the English Channel. The compacted sand was a delight to run on and, having reached the Cap Blanc Nez lighthouse, I turned back. Just then I needed to use the loo. Except there wasn't one. And barring a few fishermen, I was alone: it was the perfect opportunity to try out my sister's top tip for shaving multiple minutes from my race times. No longer would I waste time hopping from leg to leg in porta-potty queues. Not for me a frantic search for a suitable shrub followed by a furtive squat while risking mooning the entire marathon field. I was going to run like an elite runner and learn to go on the go.

At first it felt wonderful releasing the pressure from my overfilled bladder. But a second later I felt a stinging sensation between my thighs. The uric acid was flowing over the chafe I'd developed and it felt as if my legs were being eaten by ants. Then I noticed that all the pee was running into my trainers.

'Loren didn't mention *that*,' I thought grimly, trying to run with my legs wide apart while continuing to wee. It made no difference; the flow continued to course down the inside of my legs rather than becoming airborne and hitting the sand between them as I'd imagined it would. Once finished, I had something else to contend with: squelchy shoes that were rather stinky, too.

When I got back to the campsite my husband took one whiff and asked: 'What on *earth* have you been doing?'

'Trying out… a new way to… wee,' I told him between fits of giggles before hastily retreating to the ablution block where

I spent half an hour rinsing my trainers. You'll be relieved to know I never tried this particular technique again. A pee in the bush, I decided, is worth two in the shoe.

One of my most memorable 'fun runs' took place in Turin, Italy. It's not only the home of the world-famous Shroud but also the birthplace of Nutella, Cinzano and Fiat. I joined the six-hour pacing group which had two leaders whose job it was to get us to the finish line before the six-hour cut-off. This proved to be a wise move as I soon discovered that one of my pacers, a sociologist called Sue Cesarini, had an encyclopaedic knowledge of the city that had been Italy's first capital 150 years ago. She was the perfect pace-setter: moving at an ideal chat-run pace she kept our minds off the distance by regaling us with historical titbits. When we were cheered on by men in medal-festooned military uniforms wearing jaunty felt hats sporting a single black raven feather, Sue explained these were members of Italy's crack mountain-warfare troops, the Alpini, who're famous for two reasons: their ability to outfight and outgun almost anyone in the treacherous mountains, and their ability to outdrink just about anyone, too. But it wasn't just as a tour guide that Sue excelled: she also had the world's best sense of humour. Whenever we passed a refreshment station she'd wave away the water and ask if they had Martini instead (a routine that once backfired, she told me, when runners from her running club duly produced the much-requested drink and insisted she down it mid-race). And she kept asking the volunteers dishing out sponges whether they had any soaked in Chanel No 5. Having run through numerous villages with locals in traditional dress shouting *'Forza! Forza!'*, we arrived on the Corso Francia, an unbelievably long, straight road leading to the finish. I would usually have flagged by this point, but the group started singing snatches of Italian opera and when I could stop laughing long enough I joined in. Next time the going gets tough, try a touch of *La donna è mobile* to put a spring in your step. I took away two things from Turin: a new friend in Sue, and a new habit of carrying little sachets of Nutella with me as race refreshments. And, when the mood grabs me, I'll request a Martini at aid stations just for the hell of it, because Sue taught me that laughter is often much more energising than sports gels.

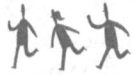

Another marathon that stands out for its sheer *joie de vivre* was the Stockholm Jubilee Marathon. This once-in-a-lifetime event was held on 14 July 2012 to mark the hundredth anniversary of the Olympic Games in Sweden – at which two of my South African countrymen (Kennedy Kane 'Ken' McArthur and Christian Gitsham) had won gold and silver in the marathon. The 2012 race was unusual. Instead of awarding prizes to the fastest runners, the top 50 best-dressed runners received awards, with the overall winner being presented with a specially commissioned medal in 18-carat South African gold worth a reported €3,000. At last I had a realistic chance of standing on the winner's podium, possibly for the first and last time in my life, so I threw myself into a frenzied search for fancy dress. I decided to go for a look that combined 'Edwardian lady spectator' and '1912 Olympic runner', so I purchased a huge orange hat decorated with feathers along with a large white T-shirt (to which I sewed a miniature South African flag) and a pair of baggy mid-calf white basketball shorts. I prayed I would look like an Edwardian and not Eminem.

At the press conference the day before I'd met a contingent of friendly South Africans who'd come to pay homage to our compatriot Ken. It didn't matter to us that he'd in fact been born in Dervock, Ireland, and had emigrated to South Africa at the age of 20. He'd run with a Springbok emblem on his chest and that was enough for us to claim him as our own. I'd bought some duty-free wine on my way to Sweden to celebrate post-race but once I got chatting to the South Africans after the formal dinner it didn't take much prodding for me to open a bottle or two. I ended up going to bed at about 3am giddy from laughing and black-tongued from imbibing a surfeit of red wine, only to wake up on race day in a state of intense confusion. I had forgotten to bring my watch and couldn't get the TV's remote control to work so I had no way of knowing what time it was. It looked a bit dark outside and I suspected I'd slept through the race. Panicking, I phoned reception.

'What time is it?' I shrieked at the desk clerk.

'10.15, madam,' he replied politely.

'In the morning or evening?' I demanded, knowing that in summer it stayed light in Stockholm until midnight.

'Ten in the morning,' came the bemused reply.

'Are you sure?'

'Yes, madam, I'm sure.'

I replaced the receiver, much relieved. The race wasn't due to begin until 13h48, the precise time the 1912 race started, so I had just about enough time to rehydrate and carbo-load at the breakfast buffet.

The atmosphere inside Stockholm's Olympic Stadium, the venue of the 1912 Games, was electrifying as all 8,000 of us lined up to parade around the athletics track before the start gun went off. In 1912, most of the field had worn white hats or knotted hankies on their heads to protect themselves from the ferocious heat. As part of the hundredth anniversary celebrations, the 2012 organisers had issued everyone with a commemorative hanky to be used as headgear or dunked in water to keep us cool.

A hundred years ago the Olympic marathon was run in temperatures that reached more than 30°C in the shade. One runner badly affected by the soaring temperatures back then was Shizo Kanakuri, who has the distinction of running the world's slowest marathon – until I went to Stockholm I thought that distinction was *mine*! After collapsing at around the 27K (16.8-mile) mark, Shizo enjoyed a glass of lemonade proffered by concerned locals before very quietly heading home to Japan. Crucially, however, he never formally withdrew from the race and in 1967, aged 75, he was invited back to finish it, logging an official time of 54 years, eight months, six days, five hours, 32 minutes and 20.3 seconds. Afterwards he quipped: 'It was a long trip. Along the way I got married and had six children and ten grandchildren.'

Despite not being chosen as a fancy-dress finalist I had a blast spending just over six hours enjoying quaint entertainment (traditional folk dancers, ladies' choirs, barrel-organ players and 100-year-old vintage vehicles) and old-school race refreshments such as lemon segments and tea. I didn't fly home with an 18-carat gold medal hung around my neck but the one I did get awarded will always bring back memories of a fun-filled day when we got to party like it was 1912.

I'm not the only one who thinks a good dollop of fun enlivens any run. Some marathons make fun their prime objective, such as the Marathon du Médoc, which I ran in September 2007. All the experts advise against drinking the night before a race, so when I heard about this event in Bordeaux, France, where drinking *during* a marathon is not only encouraged but virtually compulsory, I was intrigued. The winners are awarded their bodyweight in wine, and it's available at every 'water' station. And what wines they are! No 'glad bags' of cheap plonk here. In fact, the route map reads like a fine-wine catalogue. And the snacks? Forget sachets of gloopy gel or bananas, that's *so* nerdy sports scientist. At Médoc the race snacks consist of deli delights such as cubes of tender steak and artisan cheese.

Needless to say I didn't need to do too much persuading to round up a team of six. Driving through the quiet country lanes on race day, we all had butterflies in our stomachs (plus butterfly wings in the boot, ready to be donned at the start) at the thought of what we were about to attempt. Could we really hope to visit 23 wine stops and still finish before the race's 6h30 cut-off? I know that time limit sounds quite generous, but when you're running in scorching temperatures, zigzagging across gravel roads in order not to miss a wine stop and perhaps running less steadily because of all the wine, it can prove quite a challenge. They don't call it 'the world's longest marathon' for nothing.

The car parked, my sister and I changed into our outfits. Never one to do things by halves, Loren got a bit carried away and adorned herself with so many butterflies and flower garlands that she looked like a fluorescent Caribbean cocktail. The rest of the team's costumes were also Butterfly Ball inspired: Bridget and Kent, my two friends, dressed as ladybirds, while Aunty Rosie donned a bumble bee costume. The least colourful team member was my husband. Wearing black shorts and a greyish T-shirt that looked as if it had had a mishap in the wash, his only real concession to the theme was to sulkily pin a few paper butterflies to his back. Derisively I told him that he looked like a grub. This did not have the desired effect of shaming him into making more of an effort. He wasn't going to daub on face paint or attach any more butterflies to his outfit. He decided he'd interpreted the theme rather well, thank you, and set about looking as grubby as he possibly could.

Joining the throng at the start was like being drafted into a carnival-cum-rodeo. The theme that year was cowboys and Indians (we didn't get the memo!), so we crooned a few Country and Western songs before starting to shuffle through Pauillac's narrow streets. Suddenly we picked up the pace and everyone hurtled down a small alley to the right, heading for the first wine stop. With our first tasting under our belts, we trotted on, passing row upon row of grape-laden vineyards. The grapevines didn't offer us any shade but they did make handy privacy screens for al fresco loo visits. Dare I say we may just have rumbled the secret of the region's world-famous wines?

Racing against the clock, we had to not only reluctantly abstain from joining the locals in dancing at each wine stop, but had to overcome an even more daunting challenge: the most tempting food stalls were situated in the final few kilometres, and they slowed us down quite considerably. Mercifully, the entire Butterfly Ball succeeded in beating the cut-off, though we all posted some of our slowest-ever times. However, one record was most definitely broken that day, by the unlikeliest of competitors: my darling husband Graham, aka The Grub. At the finish line he proudly announced, to much laughter, that, unlike in Edinburgh, he'd actually rather enjoyed the race. The best bit for him? Setting a course record in oyster consumption by slurping down an unequalled 18 of them en route.

Sometimes it's the small things in a race that can provide the most mirth. Take the 2012 Malta International Challenge Marathon, a 42.2K race that's run in stages over three days. During this event I forged a friendship with two fellow back-of-the-pack runners, Antoinette, aged 65, and a 76-year-old Scotsman called Angus. The event had obviously had problems with 'bandits' (runners who race without paying for the privilege) in the past and hence the race brochure had a long section explaining that refreshments were for marathon runners only and that bandits would not be tolerated. The organisers had even gone to the trouble of issuing runners with wristbands to make sure the aid-station volunteers would only hand out water to official entrants. What made me laugh, however, was that the 'anti-bandit legislation' was all in the race brochure, which bandits would, naturally, not be issued with.

As I was chugging my way up a steep hill towards the Dingli Cliffs a few hundred metres behind Angus, unmistakeable in his tartan shorts and tam-o'-shanter, I espied several signs alerting runners to the presence of water tables ahead. When Angus reached a tiny chapel on the clifftop, he showed his wristband, grabbed a bottle of water from the table and continued up the road, only dimly aware of an oddly agitated man leaping up from the chair where he'd been dozing. Dismissing him as an overly enthusiastic spectator, Angus carried on running. However, the fellow soon caught up with him and tried angrily to wrench the water bottle back, yelling 'Euro!' Euro!' Poor Angus had mistaken a vendor's snack stand for the advertised water table just around the corner, and had inadvertently turned into a water thief not too dissimilar to the dreaded 'bandits' we had been warned about. I swear all the laughing I did that day is the reason Angus beat me. It's my story… and I'm sticking to it!

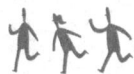

It isn't only marathons that can provide runners with more novelty value than a Christmas cracker: shorter races can come up with the goods, too. Take HellRunner, for example, a race series billed as 'off-road, off-piste and off the scale' by its organisers, where even the portable toilets have been rechristened as the suitably ominous 'Bogs of Doom'. Hell Down South, a ten-mile-ish (16K-ish) cross-country caper in Hampshire, gives you the chance to run through spooky woods with no hope in hell of knowing where you are (the absence of mile markers is deliberate) and to emerge, giggling uncontrollably, from a pit of slime with a bucketload of algae in your knickers. Having battled through it once with a fellow under-trained runner who couldn't stop swearing (no, it wasn't the celebrity chef Gordon Ramsay, although he was also competing that day), and having love-hated every second, I'm sorry to say, I won't be back. Yes, uncharacteristically I vowed immediately on finishing to do it all again (the camaraderie and home-made cake at the finish definitely had something to do with my 'all is forgiven' attitude) but I chickened out when I heard that in years past they'd had to break the ice on the water obstacles with sledgehammers before the race could start. In my book, pneumonia is too high a price to pay to scamper through puddles with people dressed in mud-splattered robes holding up signs saying: 'We're nuns with dirty habits'

A few years later, however, I did get sucked into doing another mud run. I'd read reviews of grown men being reduced to wet-pants-wearing, wobbly-kneed wrecks by the authentic-looking zombies that had pursued them through the undergrowth during the Zombie Evacuation Race. This is why I opted to be the hunter rather than the hunted. Yes, it would mean running about 500m instead of the 5K the evacuees would run but at least I wouldn't die of a heart attack.

I soon realised this was a wise precaution when I met my fellow zombies in the make-up hut. These weren't half-baked undead like me who'd written 'Ouch' in red paint on an old T-shirt and were hoping that their acting skills would get them through. No, these were zombie fanatics who actually *owned* the contact lenses that make your irises look white and who were prepared to glue dried maggots, the kind usually fed to fish, onto their hair.

My task as a zombie was to snatch the three strips of fabric attached with Velcro to the evacuees' waists: if they managed to complete the course with at least one 'lifebelt' then they'd be awarded a 'survivor' medal; the rest would get 'infected' medals. Simple, you might think, but I hadn't counted on how much the runners liked staying uninfected and hence were prepared to fight back. It was strangely amusing to growl at a wild-eyed 30-something-year-old man who begged me for mercy as he scrambled along a muddy bank, his feet failing to get any purchase on the path. But it was less funny when other runners roughly swatted my searching hands away or ganged up in groups to charge at me like enraged bulls. After one such stampede, in which I was hurled against an oil drum, I looked down in horror at my arm which was covered in huge globs of a yellow and red substance.

'No! NO!' I wailed. 'They've broken my bloody arm! Yikes! Is that what bone marrow looks like?' The only thing I couldn't work out was why I wasn't in more pain. And then I remembered. A little earlier in the course a fellow zombie had been issued with a bucket of custard and red food dye. He'd obviously done a great job in lobbing some of it at the runners – who'd then wiped it onto me. And so, I'm happy to report, I survived that little zombie apocalypse, limbs intact and funny bone tickled.

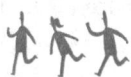

A much softer option than the Zombie Evacuation Race was the London Onesie 5K Dash, where one runs through the City of London dressed in an adult babygro. I was immediately sold when I saw the race's catchy catchphrase: 'All for onesie, and onesie for all!' and signed up on the spot. Having purchased my outfit – a pink Primark onesie with leopard-print arms – I was eager to show it off to my husband, but he most certainly wasn't as delighted with it as I was. In fact, he was horrified. He thought I looked like an 'adult baby' – the term for someone who has a fetish for regressing to an infant-like state – but I refused to be put off. I live in a freezing house with a husband who has a furnace-like metabolism. Ninety-five per cent of our arguments during our long married life have revolved around one thing: the thermostat. Don't get me wrong, unlike some people, I don't wear my onesie to the airport, or the shops. I wear it while working from home – on days when it's really cold and I don't expect any parcels to be delivered.

But I *did* wear it to the Onesie 5K Dash. This one-off charity event was held on the coldest Sunday of the year so I was very grateful to be covered from neck to toe in pink fleece. The City is pretty much deserted at 8am on weekends so, once I'd got my race number, I searched in vain for a coffee shop to warm up in, before locating a small supermarket where I took shelter. Shivering, I wandered round the aisles a few times until I found an empty pie warmer that had already been bagsied by two women wearing tigersuit onesies.

'Budge up,' I said. 'I hope you don't mind if I warm my hands, too, as my fingers are starting to turn black from the cold.'

'Not at all,' said the Tigerladies, toasting their hands in the oh-so-welcome warm air blasted into the cabinet. Our hands slowly started to thaw but all three of us agreed we were *still* cold.

'Do you think it would be rude if I climbed *into* the pie warmer?' asked Tigerlady number one. Before I could answer a shop assistant arrived with a tray of pies.

'Sorry ladies,' he said, 'I'm going to have to ask you to move as we can't have customers waving their hands over the food.'

Reluctantly we withdrew our hands, stepped away from the pies, and headed outside to join the other onesie-wearers for the start. 'Three! Two! Onesie!' shouted the starter, and then we were off, leapfrogging over bollards, swinging round lampposts and giving tourists a sight they wouldn't find in any guidebook. Onesie's for certain, not a single runner cared about their time that day – they were just too busy having a good one.

So what has running taught me about laughing? For one thing, it's an indispensable part of running – the more fun you have while running, the more you'll want to do it, no matter how tough, tiring or terrible it feels at times. 'He who laughs, lasts!' the author Mary Pettibone Poole once wrote. In fact, the renowned running author Christopher McDougall has claimed that playfulness and having fun are key to the success of many of the world's greatest ultrarunners, such as Barefoot Ted of *Born to Run* fame, Scott Jurek and Kilian Jornet. In an interview with *Men's Running* magazine he said: 'Most of us look at exercise as a terrible thing we have to endure, but Ted opened my eyes to the idea that the one foolproof way to make sure you'll always be in shape is by turning exercise into a form of play. Ted runs for fun. When it's not fun, he'll stop for a rest, have a chat, lie down in the grass. He may not get the most gruelling workout every day, but because he's having fun, he'll be back for another one.'

Laughter is also a great fear-buster. Like many newbie runners, I was afraid of making a fool of myself by running like Phoebe from *Friends*, all legs akimbo and arms waving like a wonky windmill; I was terrified of the hot-faced humiliation I was convinced I'd feel if I came last in a race. But when I let go of my ego and instead hugged my inner comedian, it gave me the courage to do things I'd never have imagined being brave enough to try: adventure racing (despite crashing my kayak and thinking I'd need stabilisers for my bike as I'd never ridden a road bike before), trail running (I frequently come last but the cake makes a great consolation prize), the Four Days Marches (the world's largest walking event where 42,000 participants walk 100 miles/160K over four days in the Netherlands), and even an Olympic-distance triathlon (where a mantra of 'noodles and beer' once stopped me drowning in the swim section). Running's taught me that it's best to be able to laugh at yourself because, as Václav Havel, the ex-president of former Czechoslovakia, once said: 'Anyone who takes himself too seriously always runs the risk of looking ridiculous; anyone who can consistently laugh at himself does not.' I guess that explains why I always run races in fancy dress – I don't want to run the risk of looking ridiculous by taking myself too seriously!

'Our funniest runs'

'The volunteer doled out sports drink like it was liquid nitrogen'

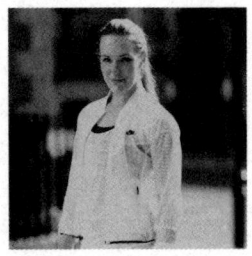

The Semi-Marathon de Paris. It'll be tough, but I'm here for a purpose: I've trained hard – and have fancy kit. Seriously, I look like I've walked off a post-apocalyptic Hollywood film set, the victorious heroine who does all her own stunts. I can't fail in my mission to run a sub-two-hour race. I refuse to.

Nearing the halfway point, the time is tight but I can do this. I'm a bit annoyed at having had to reduce my speed in the first half for people soaking up the atmosphere and high-fiving children. Don't they know THIS IS A RACE? At the fuel station, the scene is pandemonium: a mad scramble to collect fruit, water or a splash of MegaIonPowerElectroThirstAnnihilator. The volunteer 'pourer' is clearly a staunch socialist, equally dividing the rations of sports drink into small cups from a standard 500ml bottle. 'Just give me a whole one!' I shout, trying not to slow down. If you've ever attempted to get a waiter's attention in Paris then you'll know how this plays out. I am ignored and stare daggers as he carefully measures out 2.5 cups to every bottle like it's liquid nitrogen. I swipe a cup as quickly as he puts it down but miss my mouth, coating myself in sugary wetness. Now I'm faced with a hill, cobbled, covered in banana peels and 10,000 plastic cups. Is this a joke? La Comédie-Française? I scramble to the top, sliding every which-way as I go, where I am reunited with my equally traumatised running partner. This is a disaster! That cost us, what, 45 seconds? What a waste of time! We make noises to express our outrage. The noises turn to giggles, the giggles into laughter, the laughter takes our breath away, and we stop and walk, finally appreciating the hilarity of it all. I can't remember my finishing time, but because of those ridiculous 45 seconds I've never forgotten that a race is a race, but if we're not smiling, we'll never really win.

Miette L. Johnson, 33, London, England

'Nightclubbers and bikers are our running buddies in the Congo'

Trying to train for a marathon while living in the Democratic Republic of Congo is anything but a walk in the park. For a start there are no parks (and very few runnable pavements) as Lubumbashi, a southern copper-mining city, is still valiantly trying to rebuild its infrastructure after years of 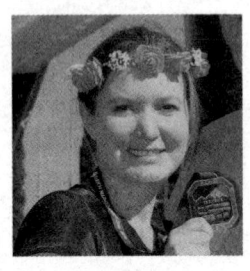 devastating civil war. Hence running on the roads themselves was the only option open to my fiancé Ernest and I when we began our preparations for the 2013 Athens Classic Marathon. In practical terms, this meant getting up at 4.30am on weekdays to do our shorter runs and 3am on Sunday mornings to fit in our 21K long run without literally running in the traffic – or the searing tropical heat. We thought that running 21K so early on a Sunday would be a somewhat lonely and cheerless affair but we couldn't have been more wrong. Far from being deserted, our route down Revolution Road was packed with revellers who'd spilled out of the nightclubs and shebeens (local beer taverns) lining the road. After recovering from the initial shock of seeing two very strangely dressed expats panting up the road in the middle of the night, several of the patrons, Simba beers still in hand, would spontaneously join us, accompanied by whoops of glee from their drinking buddies. Our newfound running companions would run behind us as best they could but, truth be told, there was a lot more bobbing and weaving going on than running. After a few metres the fact that they'd had a few too many Simbas would catch up with them and they'd stop, whereupon the revellers at the next tavern would take up where they left off.

Running before dawn did admittedly mean encountering less traffic but the downside was that we did it in near darkness. It wasn't only dark because the sun hadn't come up yet. Frequent power cuts meant the streetlights were often not working. In addition, many local motorists have a disconcerting habit of switching off their headlights every time they go downhill in the belief that it saves diesel. Having been hit by a plank lying across the back of one such near-invisible truck travelling downhill with its lights off (despite both wearing reflective belts) we realised that we needed to do more to increase our visibility, as reflective gear only works when... vehicles have their lights on! In our previous running life you could've sworn we were direct descendants of Henry Ford as we'd both buy all of our running kit in any colour as long as it was black. In a bid for greater safety and visibility on the road, however, we reluctantly retired all our beloved black gear in favour of matching Baryshnikov-esque neon tights, luminous green Nike running shoes and parrot-orange reflective tops. If this wasn't bad enough, Ernest insisted on wearing a camping headlamp facing forwards while I was told to wear mine facing backwards so that cars coming from behind could see us even if their light were off. The whole point of this elaborate get-up was to ensure that the local traffic could supposedly take steps to avoid mowing us down. But in Lubumbashi our outfits had the opposite effect. Cars that were travelling quietly down the middle of their lane would catch sight of us, switch on their brights (temporarily blinding us in the process) and then swerve straight at us to get a better view.

Despite the many and varied challenges of maintaining a running programme in Lubumbashi we've grown to love running here. Where else would you get motorbike taxis that turn around at the bottom of a hill and ride slowly (albeit on the wrong side of the road) next to you all the way back to the top with both the driver (sporting a construction hardhat instead of a helmet) and his passenger yelling '*Courage! Courage!*'?

Loren Jackson, 45, Lubumbashi, Democratic Republic of Congo

'No matter how hard we rubbed, we just couldn't get rid of the greasy stain'

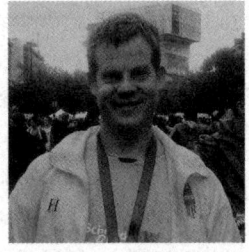

When friends coaxed me out of running retirement by asking me to run the Paris Marathon with them, I was very apprehensive: I hadn't done a marathon for 14 years since tearing a knee ligament during the London Marathon. On race day I rose super-early, conscious of the need to hydrate and carbo-load. Having dressed with the laboured demeanour of a man awaiting execution, I nervously sat down on the sofa to await my fellow runners.

After running the marathon my friends and I returned to our rented apartment in Montmartre, tired yet triumphant, only to notice a large, dark blotch on the cream-coloured sofa that none of us could recall being there before. We pondered what could have caused the stain, which resembled a Rorschach inkblot test, speculating about everything from spilled food to incontinence. Despite vigorously scrubbing the fabric with washing-up liquid and water the oily mark refused to budge and, when we came downstairs the next morning, the stain had, if anything, grown. All we could do was pray that it would dry out after we'd left and so help us avoid a costly dry-cleaning bill.

It was only when we were on the train back to London that the penny finally dropped. 'It was you!' shrieked my wife Dragana, who'd been pondering the matter all morning. The stain had indeed been caused by me: in my race-day fidgety state I'd slathered my thighs and nether regions with sufficient Vaseline to lubricate an entire tractor engine. Despite wearing three pairs of tights, the 'invisible' greasy gel had melted and seeped through my clothing like water through a sieve, leaving an unsightly imprint of my slimy *derrière*. What has now fondly been christened 'Vaseline-gate' has taught me a very important lesson: bum-printing furniture is not a good way to memorialise a race, so for goodness sake only apply the stuff *after* leaving the house!

John O'Dowd, 41, Croydon, London, England

'Being "The Back-up" is a tough job, but someone's got to do it'

Whatever you've been told, running's the easy bit. It's a simple, repetitive, one-foot-in-front-of-the-other task. All any runner really has to do is somehow make it from the start to the finish, collect a medal and receive acclamation. Easy as apple pie.

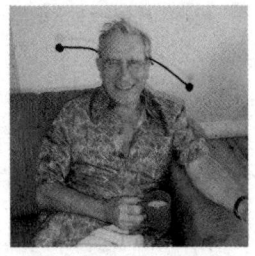

Being 'The Back-up', however, requires a good deal more. Yes, blowing up and waving balloons at various points along the route will give you a high but, remember, you'll also need to dig deep and exhibit selflessness, stamina, empathy and sympathy. You must be willing to swot up on shortcuts around towns you've never visited before – and definitely never want to visit again. You'll have to withstand driving rain and heatstroke and parking fines, not to mention be capable of completing rather tricky tasks like wheedling plastic bin liners from Bordeaux *boulangeries*

(urgently needed as emergency disposable rainwear) at 8am on race day when you speak barely a word of French. And it's compulsory that you're there to encourage your runner at the start line before racing round the course lugging a heavy backpack containing remedies for blisters, sunburn, catastrophic energy loss, creaking knees and sweaty thighs, all of which might, just might, come in handy en route. And finally, whatever you do, make very, very sure you're back in time to photograph them triumphantly crossing the finish line, find their missing clothes and carry them to the car. Oh, and did I mention you can't mind being totally ignored afterwards as your runner chats incessantly to the new friends they've made mid marathon? Fail on any of these fronts and, believe me, your future relationship could be fatally impaired. Back home, however, you'll be thanked, praised and cherished because, eventually, they'll say their success was solely due to your support. I know, because, as 'The Back-up' for my wife Rosie and niece Lisa, I've been there!

Ian 'Uncle Ian' Beach, Oxford, England

I didn't know what to expect during my first marathon in Brighton in 2011 and so Lisa kindly offered to pace me round the course. Much to my surprise, on race day she arrived sporting a gigantic chicken hat on her head. I was nervous about the race and even more so about the prospect of running 26.2 miles next to someone dressed like that. However, it wasn't long before I started to feel like a rock star as Lisa received the most cheers of anyone – the crowds absolutely loved her hen headgear. And then she stopped for a quick toilet break behind a bush. The entire seafront got a flash of her bottom and the chicken bobbing just above the foliage, and I laughed so hard I knew I'd make it through my first marathon.

Rhalou Allerhand, 35, London, England

Imagine if Rodin had sculpted the statue of *The Thinker* sitting inside a portable toilet with his running tights pulled down below his knees holding a pot of Vaseline in one hand – and his penis in the other. That's exactly what the 50 runners in the queue at the San Diego Marathon saw when one of them yanked open the door after I'd forgotten to lock it. I abhor porta-potties but before a race I always have to 'go', and also use the opportunity to lubricate every body part that's likely to chafe. I normally line the seat with loo roll and grasp my manhood to prevent it accidentally coming into contact with any nasty germs. (Yes, some would say I'm being paranoid – or even anal!) 'Oh my! Oh MY!' exclaimed the woman, holding the door open for all to see... or film. When she finally slammed it shut I sat squirming with embarrassment, waited ten minutes for my unfortunate 'audience' to disperse – and prayed I wouldn't end up on YouTube!

Lou Rhoden, 58, Chicago, USA

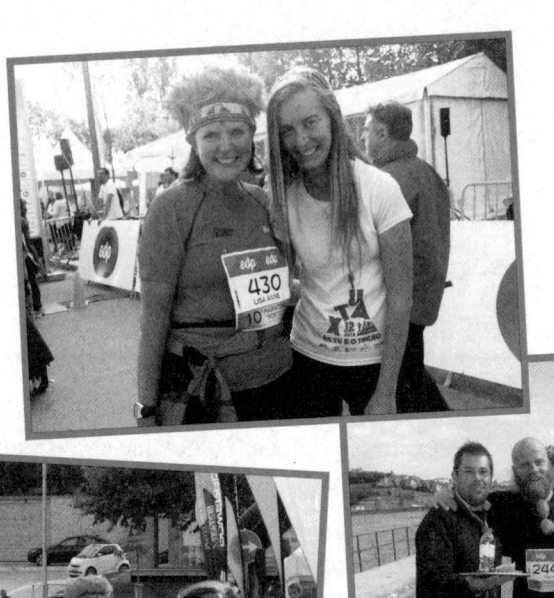

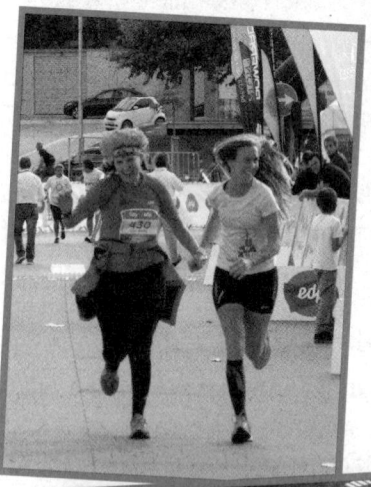

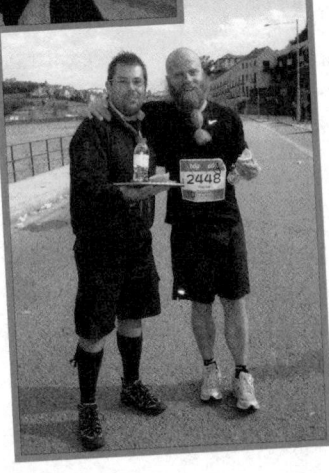

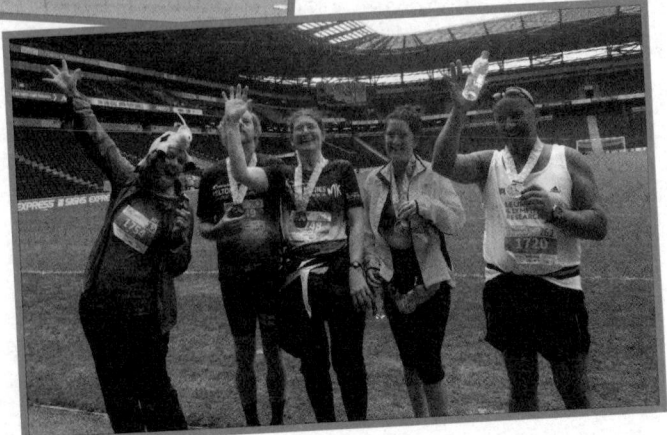

Chapter 5

What running taught me about... lifesaving

There is no exercise better for the heart than reaching down and lifting people up

John Holmes

It's Warsaw. I've got the foot of a much younger man I've known for only three hours pressed against my chest. He's begging me to push harder. I look down at him and he's writhing and grimacing in pain. Around us dozens of bemused onlookers are staring at this woman wearing a lion-head hat attempting to deliver roadside first aid to her cramp-afflicted companion. We're just 2K (1.2 miles) from the finish but the clock is ticking and if I can't get him back on his feet then we'll both go home without medals. We've run side by side for the final 20K (12.4 miles) of this marathon and made a Warsaw pact that we'd finish together. And here we are on Poniatowski Bridge, next to the spectacular National Stadium, frantically trying to stretch out his hammered hamstring. Grit from his filthy trainers is ruining my new T-shirt, but at this moment nothing matters except making sure we make it.

Someone – a good friend, actually – once called me 'The Mother Teresa of Marathon Running' because it seemed to her that nearly every time I ran I returned home with tales of limping along at the back of the pack with some poor soul who'd been on the brink of giving up for good until I took them under my wing. I've been privileged to accompany dozens of runners duelling with their inner demons and battling their own evil mental monkeys due to insufficient training, injury or advanced years. I've doled out plasters, paracetamol, chocolate, lipstick and encouragement to any runner needing it. But what my friend's Mother Teresa nickname doesn't convey is the fact that for every runner I've urged and applauded across the finish line, someone has done the same for me. Someone like John Peck, a 67-year-old former runner, who took it upon himself to become my 'bodyguard on a bicycle' during the Fort Lauderdale Marathon. John had nearly died of blood poisoning only a few weeks before after being bitten by his cat, and yet he had come out that scorching day simply to offer support to anyone needing it. He'd patiently wobbled along beside me for 18 miles (29K) (because I was running so slowly, not because he hadn't learned how to cycle properly – in fact, he's a triathlete), asking me questions and telling me stories.

Another runner came to my rescue during the 2014 Steyning Stinger Marathon in West Sussex when I got stuck in knee-deep mud with my bottom in the air in a Twister pose. As he viewed my fruitless efforts to use both hands to yank my leg out of the mire while my water bottle hung out of my mouth and I giggled uncontrollably, my saviour simply said: 'I'm not even going to *ask* you if you need help – I'm just going to help you,' pulling first my foot out of my shoe, and then my shoe out of the sludge. And then there was the time in 2015, during the 261 Women's Marathon in Majorca, where, because of an injury and operation, I'd run only three times in the ten weeks preceding the race. Having done the marathon the year before, I wasn't going to miss this truly fabulous event for anything, even if that meant suffering virtually from the start gun. On that occasion a photographer called Angel, a scooter-riding sweeper called Jesus and a spectator called Mary who walked beside me for the final 10K (6.2 miles), kept me going with their cheerful banter when every step was groan-inducing. (Yes, those were their actual names – talk about divine intervention.)

Attend any race – from a 5K charity fundraiser to a death-defying multi-day ultra – and you'll encounter a caring, sharing attitude, something we Africans call *ubuntu*. At the heart of *ubuntu* (the philosophy of African humanism) is the belief that 'a person is a person through other people', and I know this is what has inspired me to run as many marathons as I have: the chance to experience our interconnectedness in an increasingly polarised world that, sadly, often seems to have gone a little mad.

It's always fascinated me that, despite originating on a continent that's seen more than its fair share of sorrow, *ubuntu* doesn't accept that the human condition is one of individual isolation and despair. Unlike the French existentialist philosopher Jean-Paul Sartre who believed that 'man makes himself' and that 'hell is other people', *ubuntu*'s core tenet is that it is our common humanity that defines us. As Barack Obama put it in his speech at Nelson Mandela's funeral: '*Ubuntu* is a word that captures Mandela's greatest gift: his recognition that we are all bound together in ways that are invisible to the eye; that there is a oneness to humanity; that we achieve ourselves by sharing ourselves with others, and caring for those around us.'

When I look at the lengthening list of races I've completed I can barely remember my finishing time in any of them, but most of them conjure up a memory of a time when I was either rescued by another runner or did a spot of lifesaving myself, or when I shared something of myself with someone and in return was given something back. Christopher McDougall, the author of *Born to Run*, expresses this very eloquently: 'The reason we race isn't so much to beat each other but to be with each other.' Yes, there are many runners who agree with novelist Haruki Murakami that time spent alone is the greatest gift that running has to offer – 'Running in my own cosy, home-made void, my own nostalgic silence… is a pretty wonderful thing,' he once wrote – but I'm most definitely not one of them. I truly believe that you can't exist as a human being in isolation. And that there's great happiness and satisfaction to be gained by interacting with people, no matter how fleetingly.

For me running is about 'we time', not 'me time', and interestingly, a behavioural scientist at the University of Chicago has shown that I'm not alone in believing this. Her research demonstrated that everyone, whether introverted or extroverted, felt happier on days when they'd connected with more people socially. But more surprisingly (to the researcher, not to me), the increase in participants' happiness was almost the same whether they'd interacted with strangers or friends. Her conclusion? Even the bit players in our lives – those who make cameo appearances or sometimes don't even have any lines of dialogue – may influence our well-being. And boy, does running offer us a vast number of interesting bit players to choose from!

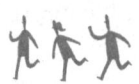

One such 'bit player' is a marshal called Rene Pilbeam, whom I met at the Beauty and the Beast Marathon. I'm not too fond of reading race websites – I simply can't be bothered with anything that makes running seem like a bit of a faff – so when I arrived at the 850-year-old Stonor House near Henley-on-Thames I was horrified when I first spotted the humongous hill facing it, which I later learned had been described as 'lung-bursting and soul-destroying' by the organisers. The hill and I soon became better acquainted when I followed the arrows pointing up it to registration and the start line. As I breathlessly ascended I heard a fellow competitor mutter: 'Blimey, if it's this hard to get to the start, imagine how tough it's going to be to get to the finish!'

At the summit I learned that the 'Beauty' referred to the gorgeous Oxfordshire countryside and the 'Beast' was a reference to the 'never-ending ascent' at the end. 'What the hell have I let myself in for?' I thought fearfully as I set off down the grassy slope after the start gun had sounded. I soon found out. While most of the other runners were charging full tilt downhill – pretty much like those you'll see chasing a seven-pound circle of Gloucester cheese if you Google 'Cheese Rolling Festival' – I was tempted to sit on my tush and slide to the bottom – the track was *that* slippery. The only problem was that almost all of the spectators had gathered at the top of the hill to watch, and I didn't want to become the event clown *too* early on.

If I'd bothered to read the website I'd have realised that the race billed itself as 'the UK's toughest multi-lap marathon' and consisted of six laps, meaning that the Beast of a hill would need to be tamed half a dozen times. But I soon discovered there wasn't just *one* Beast to conquer; there were several energy-sapping climbs – the Beast just happened to be the most savage.

At the end of lap one, having almost crawled my way to the top of the Beast, I grabbed a handful of snacks and veered left to run downhill again. Round and round the course I ran, not knowing whether to laugh or cry. Laugh, because it was all so Grand Old Duke of York, or cry, because I knew that just as soon as I'd dragged myself up that bloody hill again I'd be edging my way down it. But despite being the toughest race I'd ever done (and realising I was likely to come last from the very first step!), I never once thought of quitting, because the runners who kept lapping me never failed to pat me on the back or offer a few words of encouragement. Some even slowed down to run with me for a little while, and one, a Bulgarian chef who'd been a total stranger only ten minutes before, asked if he could give me a hug before shooting off into the woods towards the finish line.

On the final lap I encountered a 60-something marshal called Rene. She'd been sitting on a campstool doling out ladlefuls of good cheer throughout the race and, having realised I might not make the eight-hour cut-off, was now coming towards me lugging her stool with her rucksack slung over her shoulders. Despite being dressed in trousers and walking boots, she started running alongside me. 'You're going to make it,' she said encouragingly. 'You're the last runner but if you give it all you've got you'll beat the clock.'

I assured Rene I'd do my best. We scampered and stumbled down the rocky paths, through the tufty grass and into the woods, with Rene carrying my water bottle and feeding me a banana while offering me sage snippets of trail-running advice, determined to drag out every last ounce of effort from me.

At long last we reached the Beast and Rene remained at the bottom to let me revel in the glory that awaited me at the top of the hill. I clawed my way up one final time only to find the entire organising team standing in a circle cheering and clapping for me. I felt even more heroic when, a few weeks later, a running-vlogger friend confessed that, after ascending the Beast one final time, it was the closest he'd ever come to crying on camera. Don't ever let anyone tell you coming last is humiliating: in this race I'm sure it felt even better than coming first.

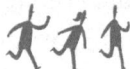

My most dramatic 'lifesaving' by far occurred during my third Beachy Head Marathon, or Bitchy for short. The first time I did Beachy I was tricked into entering by my friend Linda who told me that if I loved cake I'd love this race. And so, one Saturday in October, Linda, Belinda (who would, years later, become my beloved running buddy) and I all set off for the race near Eastbourne.

Standing at the start I looked up at the almost vertical muddy track in front of us.

'Seriously, we're not going to run up *that*, are we?' I asked incredulously.

'Oh yes,' said Linda chuckling merrily as she and Belinda shot off into the distance.

Words cannot describe how tough this event is, but I'll try. The Beachy Head Marathon is one of the most challenging trail races in the UK and has a reputation for being, well, a bitch. The course features about 3,500 feet of elevation – the equivalent of ascending an eighth of the way up Mount Everest from sea level, or climbing the Eiffel Tower three-and-a-half times. That's a solid kilometre of climbing. Whoever thought a marathon course could include 300 steps, 14 gates, several stiles and innumerable hands-on-thighs hills? And to top it all there's an up-down stretch resembling a giant crinkle-cut crisp atop the white chalk cliffs known as the Seven Sisters that's so taxing that you're tempted to go up on all fours. It's no wonder those in the know call them the Seven Bitches.

Fortunately, I met up with Lynn, who was recovering from an operation she'd undergone a few weeks before. Her wonderful tales of the unofficial running club she'd set up – the Tarts and Trouts – got me through my first Bitchy. That, plus the cake, and the sausage rolls handed out at a village aid station. (That day I learned, however, not to eat too many, as I overdid it a bit and felt a bit sick for much of the second half.)

In the car afterwards I confronted Linda: 'Er, Linda, when you invited me to do this you didn't think to mention the small matter of those rather hellish hills?'

'Look,' she said, all innocence, 'let's focus on the cake. Was it as good as I promised?'

'Yes,' I reluctantly admitted.

'Well, there you go then,' she said smiling. Case closed.

Fast-forward two years and I was back at Bitchy for the third time. This time I was dressed as a witch, as race day fell close to Halloween. It proved to be an unwise choice as my huge black pointed hat kept getting blown off by the wind sweeping in from the English Channel. Initially I ran with

Saira who was experiencing excruciating knee pain. One of our conversations involved some intriguing vegetables we'd seen growing in a field. 'Are they turnips or radishes?' we'd mused as we shuffled by. 'Let's call them radnips,' suggested Saira, 'as a turdish sounds like it fell out of a dog's bottom!'

Sadly the sweepers eventually caught up with us and said that there was no way we'd make the cut-off so we'd have to accept a lift to the finish. I told them that I had no intention of hitching a ride – and then ran my fastest Bitchy mile ever to escape them.

Afterwards Saira emailed me and said: 'Thank you for literally standing by me. It felt like we were escaped convicts – they caught up with me, but you had to keep running to avoid capture.'

My attempt to rescue Saira may have failed but I was more successful later on. On one of the Seven Sisters I came across a forlorn figure slumped on a campstool next to some coastguard trucks. By now I'd been joined by Kaz from Dagenham, who was leading a group of five marathon virgins from her running club. A runner sitting on a stool wouldn't usually worry me, but this one did: she was crying her eyes out.

'Are you OK?' I asked.

'No,' she sobbed. 'I should've pulled out at the aid station four miles back when I had the chance.'

'You probably should have,' said Kaz matter of factly, 'but you didn't. And it's too late now.'

'Yes,' I chipped in, 'now that you're at mile 20 you'd be foolish not to finish. It's just six miles. Come with us and we'll get you through.' The runner, Luisa, reluctantly joined us as we set off down yet another stone-strewn slope. After five minutes I cast a glance at her and saw that tears were still rolling down her face. I grew concerned.

'Luisa,' I said, 'I know you're hurting but you need to tell me, is the pain in your head because you're exhausted and this is the toughest thing you've ever done? Or is the pain the result of an injury? If you're injured I would *never* suggest you continue, but if you're only feeling a bit sorry for yourself – like we all are – then just listen to the stories Kaz and I are telling and forget you're even here. Before you know it you'll be at the finish line.'

Just then Kaz caught up with us, spotted the tears and spookily paraphrased exactly what I'd said.

'You see, Kaz agrees with me!' I said triumphantly.

Luisa nodded, whispering: 'It's head pain.'

'Right then, you're staying with us,' said Kaz commandingly.

On we trudged, with Kaz entertaining us with her account of how she'd lost an amazing 7 st (44.5 kg) by attending a slimming club and running, and me dusting down my funniest marathon stories to tell our bedraggled group. I was utterly amazed that the five virgins attempted Bitchy at all. 'You do know,' I told them, 'that this is one of the toughest marathons in the UK and if you can survive Beachy, any other marathon will be a doddle.'

All I got in reply were groans.

And then something rather wonderful happened. Luisa suddenly started sharing her own stories with us, becoming the life and soul of our group. It was such fun yomping along while laughing at her tales that I completely forgot about the time. When I did get round to looking at my watch I felt a knot in my stomach: it dawned on me that if I didn't get my skates on I was in danger of missing the nine-hour cut-off.

'Will you hate me for ever if I run on ahead?' I asked Kaz. 'It's just that if I don't get an official time it won't count towards my membership of the 100 Marathon Club.'

'Not at all, off you go,' she said generously. 'And don't worry about us, we're so close to the end we'll definitely finish.'

I sprinted off as fast as I could, not that anyone watching would've called it a sprint – more likely a warp-speed waddle. Fortunately, this stretch was pretty flat and I managed to pick up a fair bit of momentum. But then I came to the top of the precipitous hill we'd run up at the start. I momentarily contemplated dropping onto my bottom and descending it that way but I could see the clock reading 8:58:10 and knew this simply wasn't an option. Arms outstretched like a dive-bombing seagull I hurtled down the slope, my heart pounding like a bongo drum. As I ran full pelt across the line the clock proclaimed 8:59:59. I'd made it by *one* second!

I was being given a lift by a fleet-footed friend who'd been waiting for me for three hours so I couldn't hang around to see Luisa and 'Kaz and the Virgins' cross the line, but as I eased my aching body into the car I heard a series of whoops emanating from the finish. 'They've all made it!' I thought to myself.' They'd achieved what 90 minutes before they'd thought was impossible.

Three years later Luisa, the woman who'd sat crying on a campstool, finished a half Ironman triathlon. And then she did another one. And now, I hear, she's training for a full Ironman-distance triathlon, a feat that involves swimming for 2.4 miles (3.9K), cycling for 112 miles (180K) and then running a marathon. So it seems that the philosopher Nietzsche was right after all: what doesn't kill you does make you stronger.

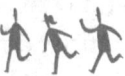

Interestingly, as you may have guessed, it's often not easy to distinguish between who's the rescuer and who's being rescued. As I've discovered time and time again. The 2015 Milton Keynes Marathon was a case in point. Having been diagnosed with bruised bones, plantar fasciitis and tendonitis (yes, all at once), which basically translates as 'flipping sore feet', I was having a tough time of it. Until, that is, I met Vivien and Charles who, though power-walking, somehow managed to keep passing me. We hitched up at mile ten when Vivien was almost in tears because she feared not beating the 6h30 cut-off. One of the best things about marathon running is feeling that you're in the position to help another runner reach the finish line. 'If you can bear my incessant chatting,' I told her, 'I can guarantee you'll make it.' And so, with Charles acting as our timekeeper, we pressed on, sharing sweets, chocolates and stories. I never found out what ailed Vivien that day, as to ask her would've reminded her to focus on it, but there were times when I'm convinced she was crying.

'Charles is making me nervous when he says "uh, oh" every time he looks at his watch at the mile markers,' she said.

'He's keeping us on pace so we need to be grateful to him for that,' I said, jog-trotting next to her as I couldn't quite keep up with her speedy walking pace.

Just then we stumbled across Jemma, a 23-year-old marathon first-timer who was clearly not having a good time.

'I'm never, ever, *ever* going to do another marathon,' she vowed at mile 19.

'Oh, everyone says that at the finish,' I laughed.

'Well, I'm saying it *now*,' she muttered through gritted teeth.

'Tell me that again after you've slept with your medal on,' I replied. 'You're 23. Twenty-three! How many other women your age do you know who've done a marathon? You are going to be *soooo* proud after this – it's an achievement no one can ever take away from you.'

Stephen was the next runner to join our band of brothers. He was running in honour of a friend who'd died of leukaemia at the age of 55. There truly is strength in numbers and it felt so good to be part of a group, all running for our own different reasons, each dealing with their own personal issues, all egging each other on. With six miles to go, Vivien picked up the pace and so the challenge now lay in not losing sight of her. I alternated between checking on her up front and slowing down to make sure Jemma didn't get left behind. When Stadium MK appeared Vivien shouted: 'We're going to make it!' and thanked me for giving her something else to focus on other than how much further we had to go.

'I didn't do anything other than chat to you,' I said. 'Actually, come to think of it, it's been *you* leading the way for the past six miles.'

'Yes,' she said after a short, thoughtful pause, 'but if you hadn't been here today, I wouldn't have had anyone to lead!'

With just over five minutes to spare, Vivien, Charles and I crossed the line holding hands, with Jemma and Stephen following 100 metres behind. A few days later I got an email from Stephen: 'Nothing brings people together like a marathon

– it brings out the best in us,' he wrote. 'There is no way I would have left Jemma at the last mile even if it meant not getting a medal. And yet I did not know her till then. It just shows how we can all help one another in times of hardship and it restores my faith in the human race.'

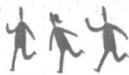

If there's one race that stands out for me as a truly international rescue effort, it's Portugal's Porto Marathon. Despite the fantastically scenic route along the Douro River I was finding it hard going, especially once the British, Italian and Swedish runners I'd met early on had surged ahead along with the entire marathon field. It was my seventh marathon in two months and the heat wasn't helping, so I was overjoyed when, at the 25K (15.5-mile) mark, I hitched up with a Dane called Bjarke, who sported the most fabulous plaited Viking-like beard. Chat-running got us through the next 6K until he suddenly ground to a halt. 'Can you get me a banana?' he pleaded. 'I saw some discarded ones on the road.'

'I'll try to find one,' I promised. Scanning the gutter I was jubilant when I found half a banana, skin intact, and offered it to Bjarke, assuring him that I'd washed the exposed cut end.

'No thanks,' he said, his eyes glazed. I offered him a gel, but this he also refused. Even the volunteer who hurried over like a silver-service waiter to offer him a bottle of water and orange segments on a tray couldn't get Bjarke to eat or drink anything.

'You really do need to get some sugar inside you if you're going to continue,' I said.

By this time Bjarke had been joined by his girlfriend who'd come to support him, and he sat down heavily on some steps.

'I'm going to have to leave you,' I said reluctantly. 'I've simply got to make it before the six-hour cut-off. But you really should try to get going again, it's just over seven miles to the finish.'

Heading off on my own I was soon joined by Ashley, an American tourist who'd decided to go for a Sunday jog along the river.

'Are you in some kind of race?' he asked, looking around for the other competitors.

'Yes, it's a marathon, but I'm the second-last runner so everyone else is ahead of me,' I laughed.

'Who's behind you then?'

'A Danish runner called Bjarke, but I don't think he's going to make it as he's really out of it. His blood sugar's rock bottom.'

'Would you like someone to run with?' Ashley asked.

'That would be fantastic, I'd love the company. But if you really want to help someone out today you should go and see how Bjarke is faring and run with him.'

'OK, I'll stick with you for a bit and then I'll try to find him.'

We caught up with Elisa, a marathon newbie from Lisbon, and Ashley ran with us for a while before heading back in search of Bjarke. Elisa was just as engaging a companion as Bjarke and Ashley had been and I was immensely grateful for her companionship, especially when a driver pulled up and started shouting at us in Portuguese. 'He told me the race is over and we might as well pack it in,' Elisa said. 'And I told him to get lost.'

'Good for you! Why on earth do people who don't run think it's acceptable to be abusive to those who do?' I spluttered.

At long last we saw the red carpet leading up to the finish

line and crossed under the arch hand in hand, arms held high. 'We did it!' she yelled. 'I've finished my first marathon!'

After hugging almost everyone in sight, we turned to cheer those we'd passed in the final kilometres. Looking anxiously at the clock I feared Bjarke was going to run out of time. One minute before the cut-off the race director walked out onto the red carpet and all the volunteers gathered round to applaud him, hollering and slamming their hands against the metal hoardings lining the last 100 metres of the course. Beaming, and visibly moved by their cheers, the race director wiped a tear from his eye. But who was that behind him? I barely dared look. It was none other than bearded Bjarke, flanked by Ashley and a handful of volunteers who'd dashed onto the course to bring him home.

'Come on! Come on!' I shouted. 'Hurry up! You can do it!'

And you know what? Bjarke did. In one of the most nerve-wracking finishes I've ever seen, and with just five seconds to spare, he crossed the finish line where a TV crew were anxious to interview him. By the time he was ready for his hug I'd blown my nose and wiped at least some of the tears I'd shed at his triumph from my face. It had taken a veritable League of Nations – a Brit, an Italian, a Swede, a Dane, an American and a Portuguese runner – to rescue my race. That day in Porto, I really did see the old Zambian proverb in action: 'If you want to go fast, go alone; if you want to go far, go together.'

But running hasn't just taught me about the kind of lifesaving we all do when we take the time to help another runner reach the finish line. Spending time with those runners has made me aware that running itself can be a lifesaver. In my case, achieving running feats I once believed to be impossible led to me having the courage to tackle other major challenges, such as becoming a writer at the age of 36 and retraining as a clinical hypnotherapist at the age of 40. These are two incredibly rewarding careers and I now have a day job where I can categorically say I can make a difference. Running has, quite literally, saved me from spending the next 20 years feeling unfulfilled professionally. And I'm not unique in having had this experience. Time and again I've been told how the simple act of putting one foot in front of the other has helped people overcome addiction, depression and low self-esteem. Running has enabled them to end bad relationships and forge new ones. I would never have met the extraordinary runners whose stories you're about to read below if I hadn't become a runner, and my life has been immeasurably enriched by knowing them. In their own way, each of them is an inspiration. Whenever I line up at the start of a race I wonder whom I'll encounter that day. While the race website may advertise that each runner will receive a medal, T-shirt and goody bag, I know that I'm likely to come away with things that are a lot more precious – new friends. But also something else. A continued belief in the rather miraculous redemptive power of running.

'Running was my lifeline'

'I ran towards the rest of my life and left my old one behind'

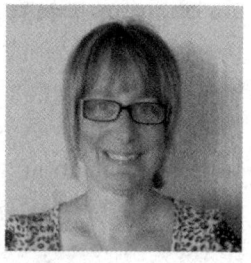

In 2008 my Dad passed away suddenly and my marriage broke down. One of the things that helped me through this difficult time was running. I hadn't entered a marathon before but when a friend asked me to do the Beachy Head Marathon with her I leapt at the chance. I found the training hard but it made me focus on something other than my sadness.

Race day was wonderfully sunny and I can't really explain in words what a fantastic experience I had. I wasn't a front runner by any means – more of a backmarker – but I do recall having a *moment* at a certain point during the marathon. I was running down a hill and I felt I was running towards the rest of my life and leaving my old one behind. I knew that if I could finish this marathon I could cope with anything life could throw at me – I can still recall that feeling today.

The next year I persuaded my twin sister to join me and we raised over £3,000 for a charity our Dad was a trustee of. The torrential rain did nothing to dampen our spirits – we both carried a photo of our Dad in our pockets and knew he'd have been extremely proud of us both.

Because this marathon has a special place in my heart I've run it every year since 2008, and in 2010 met Lisa at mile eight when I ran it despite having had a minor operation a few weeks before. Whenever I reach that point where I had my moment I look back at how my life has changed and smile. I subsequently married a wonderful man who told me when we first met that I'd never get him running. He's just completed his tenth marathon.

Lynn Sims, 48, Lydd, Kent, England

'Running kept the horror of depression at bay'

Everyone needs a hobby. A little something they can lose themselves in. For me, running is it. At 34, I decided I was going to run away... literally, as if in search of something. I'd recently given up a part-time marketing job to take care of my three children under five, but instead of this making things easier I felt lost, and a little suffocated. I was also in a 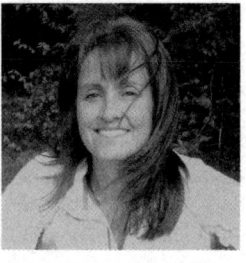 very unhappy relationship. It was while on a family holiday in Scotland that I decided to go for a run. I asked my Dad to accompany me on his bike, and when I arrived back home beaming, feeling refreshed and alive again, I realised this was going to be big. I started training regularly and began discovering the beautiful area I live in. At times running felt like a real lifeline and kept the horrors of depression at bay.

The next step was training others: first a few mums from the playground and later paying clients, after I qualified as a personal trainer. Eventually I ended up tutoring for England Athletics. While on the outside I appeared confident, my turbulent relationship was leading to deep feelings of inadequacy. Now, for the first time in a long time I could say I was good at something – I was actually inspiring people. After much soul-searching I separated from my partner and supported myself and my children through the money I earned from being a running coach. It obviously wasn't all plain sailing but my running-club girls, the FittBirds, were amazingly supportive. I continue to enjoy training in a really stunning corner of Hertfordshire, where my late father grew up and spent his life roaming through the countryside. Running has given me a real sense of belonging here – as if I'm a part of it and it's a part of me.

Suzy Fitt, 48, Welwyn, England

'Running marathons at 81 helps me fight old age'

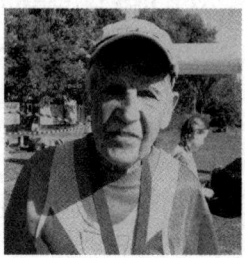

I got fat drinking up to 15 pints a day, and if I hadn't discovered running I'd be dead today, no doubt about that. Thirty-four years ago, when I was my cricket club's membership secretary, I spotted someone in the clubhouse I didn't recognise and went over to ask him to pay his dues. As I walked towards him I realised to my horror that the bloke with the stomach sticking out was me reflected in a mirror. It really frightened me, so the next day I staggered round a five-mile race at my son's running club, all the while feeling as though I was going to have a heart attack. Afterwards, however, I felt rejuvenated and decided to join the club. The next year I did myself proud with a time of 3h48 in the London Marathon. Running soon became a huge part of my life so I stopped drinking and lost 5 st 7 lb (35 kg). I also started doing ultras and travelled the world running 446 marathons with my 100 Marathon Club mates.

My nickname of Red Hat Robbie comes from the red beanie I always wear – I have ten now but I've washed them so often they've gone pink. Now I'm 81, I'm fighting old age all the time by walking everywhere, working in my allotment and continuing to run 5K parkruns (I've just done my hundredth) and the odd marathon. I've started using a stick to get around the courses without tripping and have to admit I have problems getting over stiles in cross-country races. But, as a former London jive champion, I still delight in showing off my dance moves by jiving with the refreshment-table volunteers in marathons.

Robbie Wilson, 81, Wallington, England

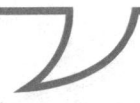

'I ran for 24 hours on a treadmill to celebrate surviving leukaemia for 26 years'

At the age of 24 I was diagnosed with leukaemia and told there was only a 50/50 chance of treatment being successful. What followed was a week of gruelling chemo and radiation therapy and then a bone-marrow transplant. I also suffered from agonising shingles as my immunity was compromised.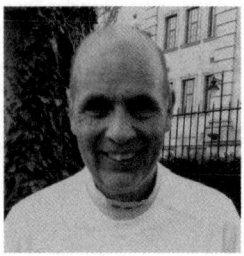

I never really thought about not making it, although there was a time when I very calmly told a doctor I'd had enough of the constant pain and didn't want to live any more. He simply replied that the pain would eventually stop, which thankfully it did.

I did my first marathon three years later, and have been racking them up ever since. Initially I wanted to break four hours, but after I did so in my third attempt with a time of 3h50 I no longer wished to run faster and now enjoy being at the back seeing other people living their dreams. Last year I was the sweeper at the Farnham Pilgrim Marathon in Surrey for the fifth time and it was immensely rewarding helping Lisa and four other runners who'd got lost find their way to the finish to ensure they got their medals. When I turned 50 I wanted to do something different to celebrate having beaten my illness, so I decided to run for 24 hours on a treadmill and raise funds for leukaemia research. I ended up doing 123 kilometres. Sleep deprivation didn't come into it, probably because I was so excited to be raising over £6,500. I'm now aiming to join the 100 Marathon Club and will also use running my hundredth marathon as a way to fundraise again. I hope it'll show people who've just been diagnosed with cancer or are going through treatment that there is hope for them to have a long, healthy and fruitful life.

John Applebee, 50, Aldershot, England

'My life fell apart when I could no longer run — but then my camera saved me'

My running career started properly at 40 when I began running at lunchtimes while teaching at a high school. Having joined a club, I began setting PBs — including a 2h34 in the Potteries Marathon just before turning 50. On the strength of these times I achieved my greatest running honour: 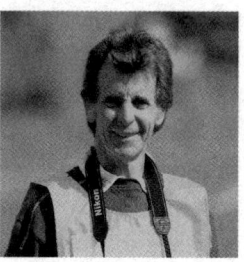 representing England in a cross-country international, where our team won gold.

Unfortunately, my racing career came to an abrupt, unhappy end. While training I tore the cartilage in my left knee so badly that I never raced seriously again. Not being able to run meant my life fell apart. Most of my friends were runners and I could no longer meet up to train and race with them. And without the stress relief that running gave me I felt unable to continue in my job as head of maths and so asked to be demoted, which was a big blow financially.

My life changed dramatically, however, when I stumbled across a race-photographs website and thought: 'I could do that.' It was the key I needed to get back into the sport I desperately missed. So I set up racephotos.org.uk, a website offering free race photos, and in my wildest dreams never thought that it would become so popular — so far it's had 1.8 million hits! Runners often shout their thanks to me as they run past, and I was thrilled to be nominated to carry the Olympic Torch in 2012. I still get out for a slowish, shortish run most days: when the old lady with the Zimmer frame passes me, perhaps then I'll call it a day!

Bryan Dale, 73, Staffordshire, England

'Being blind spurred me on to run over 250 marathons'

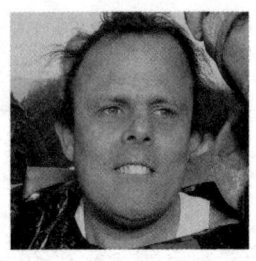

I lost my sight at the age of six due to hydrocephalus (fluid on the brain) and at seven was sent to a boarding school for the blind where I discovered I loved running. Aged 18, I was knocked down by a car and it was while lying in a hospital bed that I made a pledge to myself that one day I'd run a marathon to prove to the medical staff that they'd done a fantastic job in mending my broken leg. Little did I know what was to follow.

Once I'd run my first London Marathon in 1989 I decided to do multiple marathons as I loved making new friends and getting out into the fresh air in places I might otherwise not have visited. I was also keen to prove that being blind was not a barrier – the only limits in life are the ones you put on yourself.

I do have some vision so can just about make out trees and hedges and people up ahead of me. My (human) guide and I use a dog's rubber toy to keep us connected. It's a figure-of-eight shape and is covered in white tape so it can be seen in the dark during the winter. Having put my trust in other people for such a long time in everyday life it's not too difficult to trust someone to guide me; in fact, the nerves are usually my guide's, not mine. I love making onlookers smile by joking: 'Don't worry, I'll get her round.' If I trip it usually causes just a minor problem like a cut leg or a sore hand. I get up and carry on as though nothing has happened and by the time I've finished any pain has usually worn off. My worst fall was during a marathon in Taunton. I tripped on the kerb and broke four ribs when I hit the bollards in the middle of a traffic island.

There have been some very good times in my running career and I've run in 15 different countries ranging from America to Lebanon and of course Greece, the home of marathon running. Becoming a member of the 100 Marathon Club at the age of 34 was a real milestone. I did my hundredth in 1999 and many of the club members took turns running with me. Just a short way from the end one person ran ahead and shouted instructions to me so that I could run across the finish line unaided. Another highlight was doing the Potteries Marathon in Stoke-on-Trent, where I got to meet the starter, the legendary footballer Sir Stanley Matthews, whose 80th birthday coincided with my 80th marathon. My 150th, 200th and 250th marathons were also all special as they were reached within the time targets I'd set myself. I wanted to get to 150 before the age of 40 but did it so quickly that I felt compelled to up that to 200!

Marathons aside, there is one very short run in 2012 that meant a lot to me. I was only supposed to do 300 metres but, the way the route was laid out, I ended up running about 1K. Most of this was in the grounds of a local college in Hereford. The run/walk was unforgettable as I was carrying the Olympic Torch. It was wonderful being honoured for what I'd achieved.

I'd like to carry on running as long as my body will let me. I aim to do between 10 and 20 miles a week on the road but often have difficulty finding people to train with.

I've now done 276 marathons and my next target is to reach 300 before the start of the 2016 Rio Olympics. Running marathons has transformed me: in a strange way I'm grateful to be blind as I very much doubt I'd have achieved everything I have so far if I wasn't.

Paul Watts, 50, London, England

'I lost my job, marriage and sister in the same year'

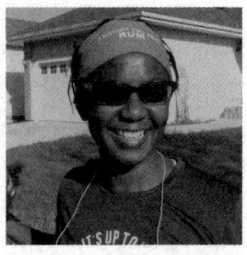

I haven't always been a runner. At the age of 35 I lost my job of seven years and my marriage of 12 years and embarked on being a single parent of two. Soon afterwards I lost my sister, and inherited her four orphaned children. I found it really hard raising six kids and working full-time, so sleeping became my only respite. I was sinking into depression but I didn't know it. When one of my friends visited she always found me asleep. Concerned, she suggested I accompany her to the gym. 'I'm already utterly exhausted, how in the world would I manage that?' I replied.

But one day she came to visit with a 'take no prisoners' attitude. 'I need ten minutes in the gym with you,' she said. 'After that you can come home and go right back to sleep.' My friend made me walk on the treadmill for ten minutes and, true to her word, we came back after that. She came the following day and the next... and gradually the ten minutes became 15, then 20. When I got to 30 minutes I realised I was faster than when I'd started – I was actually running. I began feeling more optimistic and before I knew it I'd caught the running bug big time.

I did my first marathon aged 40 – and the rest is history. Along with 20 marathons I've run the 91K Comrades Marathon in South Africa three times (which is where I met Lisa).

During some of my darkest moments I didn't want to show weakness to my children, who needed my strength to feel secure, so I'd run away from home and keep running until I could handle coming back. I run because it's cheaper than therapy, but most of all I run because it saved my life.

Mwaka Kaonga, 50, Winnipeg, Canada

It took me 25 years, 11 months and 20 days to lose my virginity – my marathon virginity, that is. That's how long it took from deciding to run a marathon on my twenty-fifth birthday to actually doing one, aged 50, because I had to lose 120 lb before I could embark on the training. I was never afraid of the distance as I'd been through worse: my son's drug addiction, my first husband's suicide. Surprisingly, it wasn't the injuries that almost sidelined me; it was trying to do everything – kids, work and my training – without asking anyone for help. I was exhausted and in pain. Then my husband John, a runner, started coaching me and leaving me encouraging notes and gel sachets along the roadside. This taught me that you have to let your family, friends, colleagues and fellow runners support you to get to the finish line. It made me start looking for ways to help others achieve their dreams, too. The marathon made me a better runner, yes, but also a better wife, mom and friend.

Nancianna Clonan, 51, Soldotna, Alaska, USA

The London Marathon was one of the toughest battles of my life and it was great to see how proud my family were of me afterwards. The true impact hit me, however, when my sister sent me a photo of Heroes Day at her daughter's school, where the children dressed up as their hero (usually famous people or book characters). The photo showed my niece wearing my running vest, London race number and a replica medal – because I was her hero. That made me cry then, and does even now.

Sally Newman-Russell, 47, Southend, England

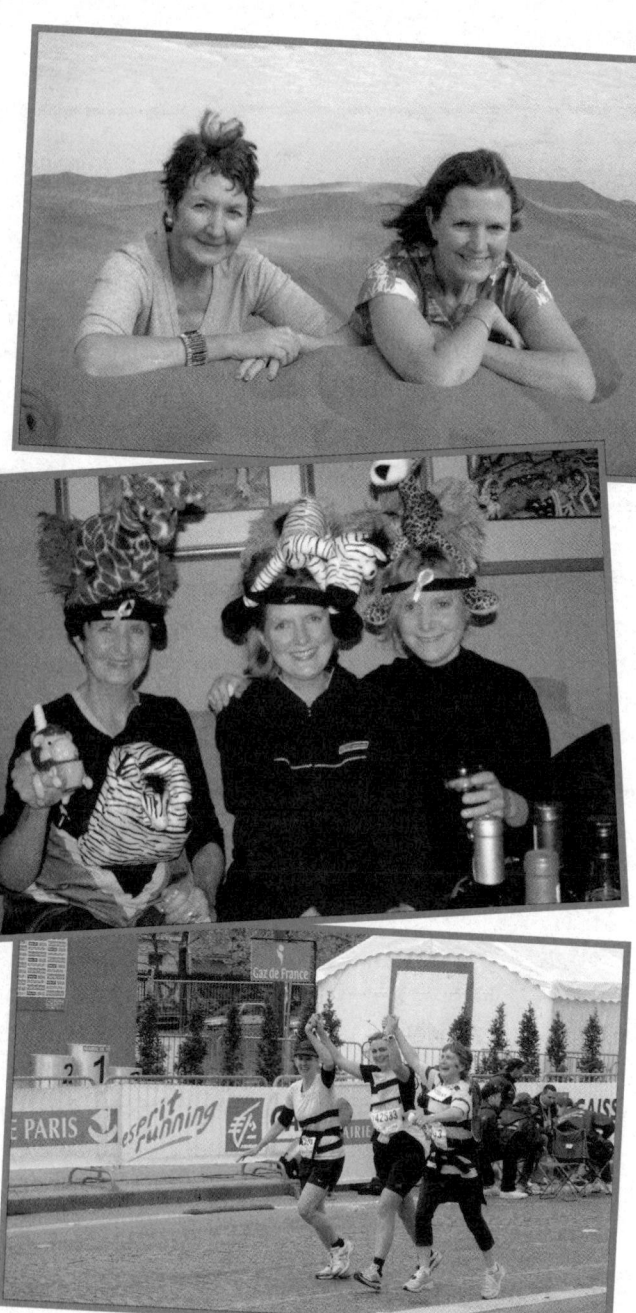

Chapter 6

What running taught me about... death

> " Our dead are never dead to us, until we have forgotten them "
>
> George Eliot

I've always thought it somewhat strange that the most life-affirming sport I know has historically always been closely associated with death. When I ran the Athens Classic Marathon in 2010 the route took an early detour around the mound where the 192 Athenians slain during the Battle of Marathon are buried. I felt very emotional realising that, 2,500 years after they'd died, we were paying our respects to the fallen in the most heartfelt way we knew – with our feet.

Later in the race we passed the statue of Pheidippides, the messenger who collapsed and died after racing from Marathon to Athens to announce the Athenian victory over the invading Persians. His epic journey and famous last words – 'We are victorious!' – continue to inspire marathon runners the world over.

For me, running will forever be associated with death not because of the Pheidippides legend but because it deprived me of my beloved mother, who was killed while training for a marathon. And because it will always remind me of Aunty Rosie, who ran eight marathons with me before she was snatched away by cancer. What I learned from both losses was that the grief you feel is in direct proportion to the amount of love you felt. It's a truly terrifying equation when you think about it – let alone experience it.

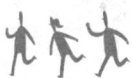

I wish you could've met my Mum. She was larger than life and, as my Dad put it, 'She had more enthusiasm in her little finger than all of us put together.' Whether it was researching religion, history, architecture or art, going to the theatre (she once saw 18 plays during a two-week trip to London) or helping the needy, she did everything with a contagious passion. She's the only woman I know who could boast of taking up marathon running and going bungee jumping, white water rafting and microlighting – all after the age of 60.

At her celebration (we never referred to it as a funeral) in 2007, held on a sunny winter's day in our garden in Pretoria in South Africa in the shade of a towering Cuban palm tree, I spoke about the Mum I'd known. I said my entire life was a testament to her. And that whereas other children might inherit material things, I had *already* received the greatest inheritance of them all: an interest in, well, just about everything. My love of literature, travel, opera, ballet (and yes, ice cream) had all been inspired by her. But my most treasured inheritance, by far, is my love of running. Not only did my Mum lead by example when she took up running in the 1970s – even if it took me two decades to follow it – but she shared all my triumphs with me, too. Throughout my running career the first person I'd phone to inform I'd got another medal was my Mum. From a call box in Princes Street I excitedly phoned her to share the news that I'd just run every step of the way in the Edinburgh Marathon. From a payphone in Berlin I related the emotion I'd felt running through the Brandenburg Gate. From Rome I rang to tell her of the PB I'd achieved sprinting past the Colosseum while wearing the same giraffe headdress I'd worn while doing the New York City Marathon with her two years previously.

Sadly, New York was one of the few races my mother and I ever ran together as 6,000 miles separated her home in Pretoria and mine in London. Mind you, when I say 'together' I mean we started out at the same time – I was always trailing in her wake. Our trip to New York came about as a result of my mother getting breast cancer at the age of 61. My sister Loren, who lived close to her, sprung into action and got her the best nutritional advice money could buy. Out went the ice cream, pizza and liquorice and in came juicing and steamed vegetables. My Mum didn't take kindly to this but she was utterly determined to get well so she juiced with a vengeance, once drinking so much carrot juice that her skin turned orange. And as for vegetables, she had two catchphrases: 'I hate 'em, but I ate 'em' and 'Vegetables? Yuk!'

When I flew out to South Africa after her mastectomy I was amazed by my Mum's positivity. She even turned wig-buying into a hilarious occasion, insisting on trying on a platinum blonde number rather than the ones that resembled her real hair.

'Mom, the wig is supposed to *disguise* the fact the chemo's made you lose your hair, not make it obvious you have,' chuckled my sister.

'I know,' she said, 'but I've always wanted to be blonde and this is the best chance I'll ever get.'

We went home with a brunette wig but, if Loren and I hadn't been there, we've no doubt that my Dad would've been looking at the prospect of being married to Marilyn Monroe for six months. In the event my Mum's hair never fell out, so the wig remained unworn, and she sailed through chemo, much to everyone's surprise.

Loren and I decided that our mother needed an inspiring goal to aim for after her chemo was over, so naturally we chose the biggest, brashest marathon on the planet: New York. My Mum was overjoyed when, as her last chemo session drew to a close, she learned that she'd got a place through the ballot. Sadly my sister and I didn't get in so we both vowed to try again the following year and deferred my Mum's place. In the event, this delay proved fortuitous: the Twin Towers were attacked that year and although the marathon went ahead, it was a very sombre occasion and not the celebratory one we'd had in mind. The following year we once again failed to get ballot places, but then my ever-generous Dad stepped in and offered to pay for us to get guaranteed (and much more expensive) places through a sports-tour company. When we arrived in New York that November, it was utterly freezing, but that didn't deter my mother who, never having been there before, set about seeing every single sight the city had to offer. The Empire State Building. Central Park. Times Square. Grand Central Station. The stuffed toys that inspired Winnie-the-Pooh. Even Ground Zero, where we paid a very emotional visit and read all the messages of remembrance that were still pinned to a nearby fence. Just about the only time we were off our feet was the terrifying five minutes we spent aboard a helicopter swooping over Manhattan.

The day before the race our feet were throbbing so much that my sister and I had to call it a day at 3pm and head back to our hotel. Not my Mum. Despite a nasty head cold, she'd insisted on touring the Metropolitan Museum of Art, finally returning at 8pm just when we were about to call the police.

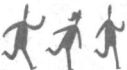

New York was one of the toughest marathons I've ever run. Not only did our overzealous sightseeing mean my feet were killing me long before we even crossed the start line, but it was brain-freezingly cold. Thankfully, we'd bought animal-print beanies and gloves to match our African-animal headdresses, but even still the Arctic winds blowing off the Hudson River weren't kept entirely at bay. My sister and I were both woefully undertrained and underprepared. I'd forgotten my sports watch, so we had to time our walk/run sections using my alarm clock – until I dropped and broke it at 13K (8 miles). Lacking the discipline the clock had given us, our walk breaks became longer and longer.

Our mother ran an entirely different race, trotting merrily along just ahead of us, pausing only to blow her nose once in a while, and to climb up a fire engine to pose for photos with some hunky firemen. She got a huge kick whenever anyone shouted out 'Go, Crazy Hat Ladies!' and revelled in the frenzied support we were greeted with when we exited the Queensboro Bridge. We crossed the finish line in Central Park in the dark in a time of 6h01. My Mum was disappointed that we hadn't finished in under six hours, not realising that running 26.2 miles at the age of 63 following a breast-cancer diagnosis only 20 months previously, while footsore, freezing and suffering from a cold, was no mean feat.

Five years later I invited my Mum to run another marathon with me. I duly began some sporadic training while my mother threw herself into hers, determined to keep up with her daughters and do us proud.

And then I got the call that would change my life for ever. I was on a press trip to Jordan when our tour leader drew me aside and said someone from work wanted to speak to me. I'd left copious handover notes before departing so I was annoyed that my colleagues should think it necessary to hassle me while I was abroad. Except it wasn't my boss on the phone, it was my Dad.

'Mommy's been killed,' he said, his voice breaking. It felt as if the entire room was drawing away from me, like the sight of the earth from a rocket surging into space. For a moment I couldn't comprehend what my father was saying. It was as if I'd entered a parallel universe in which all the normal rules didn't apply. I still wanted to hear all about my mother's recent trip to Russia. I'd expected to be running marathons with her into her eighties. I didn't want to be a motherless child at 39.

I had to sit down as a dark dread slowly filled my heart. Coming from crime-blighted South Africa, I immediately assumed my mother had been murdered. 'She was run over while out running,' my Dad continued. Relief flooded over me. My mother hadn't been tortured. She hadn't suffered. She hadn't died scared. We took great comfort from the fact that she'd been hit from behind and so hadn't seen it coming. She'd had a truly good death as she'd died while still in her prime, without experiencing ageing's slow decline into infirmity.

I flew back to South Africa and was met by a grief-stricken Loren, who'd had to identify our mother's body at the morgue. My younger brother Mark and I wanted to go to the funeral home to say our last farewells too, but Loren strongly advised us not to.

'Mom looks terrible, she doesn't even have lipstick on,' she said.

'That's not a problem – we'll take some along and put it on for her,' I said.

'You don't understand,' she sobbed. 'She doesn't… have… any lips.'

And then the full horror of what had happened hit me. A truck had failed to stop at a stop sign and had hurtled into fast-moving traffic, causing another vehicle to veer out of control, mount the pavement and mow my mother down.

In the end Mark and I went anyway. Since my sister's visit the undertakers had done an amazing job: my mother didn't look nearly as bad as I'd imagined and we were able to talk to her and touch her.

A few days later my sister and I wrote letters to the drivers involved in my mother's death. We told them that we bore them no ill will, as that's what my mother, a committed Christian, would have wanted. It was hard to write those letters but little did we know that the forgiveness we extended would actually be a gift, not to the drivers, but to ourselves. I generally find it difficult not to obsess about being wronged by others but the letters meant that I've been able to spend the past eight years entirely free of anger. Nelson Mandela was right when he said on being set free after 27 years in jail: 'I knew if I didn't leave my bitterness and hatred behind, I'd still be in prison.' He realised, as I have since, that resentment is like drinking poison and then hoping it will kill your enemies.

Finally, my memories of my mother's butterfly-themed celebration: the organist at the crematorium saying to us that 'Christian funerals are very different to other funerals because for the departed it's like graduation day'; and placing a lipstick on the top of my Mum's coffin, having put her favourite running shoes inside it (we almost included her two marathon medals but then decided they were too precious).

My Dad set the tone for the celebration when he said, 'Let's celebrate the extra seven years we had with your Mom after she got cancer, rather than the 15 or 20 years we won't get to spend with her.' And my mother, too, contributed inadvertently to the celebratory air through an email that she'd sent me several years before. The message had contained her funeral wishes, including a poem she wanted read out during the ceremony. She'd put its name in the subject line of her email, but because it had been a very long name, it wouldn't all fit into the box. 'Do Not Stand at My Grave and Wee,' my mother had, in all innocence, apparently instructed me. And so, on the saddest day of my life, I related this story with a very big smile and faithfully vowed to do as she had bade me. I had promised to neither wee – nor weep – at her grave.

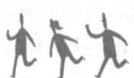

The loss of my aunt just four years later hit me almost as hard as the death of my mother. After completing our first half marathon together in Newcastle she'd run beside me in eight marathons. Aunty Rosie was a dream running companion and we'd save up stories to tell each other during our races as we both subscribed to the running philosophy that the more you talk, the faster you run. We even wore the same running shoes: Nike Vomeros, which we jokingly referred to as our Vomiteros. I always marvelled at her cheerfulness as she never once moaned about anything while running, no matter how much pain she was in. I also admired her stamina and ability to encourage not only me but other back-of-the-pack runners, who frequently mistook her for my sister.

A highlight from our many marathon exploits was finally persuading her, after seven marathons where she'd been cheered only as 'Fairy's Friend', to run in fancy dress. She ran as a bumblebee for the first time in the Paris Marathon – and applied so much yellow face paint that she ended up looking more like Marge Simpson than a bee.

And then, in February 2011, when I called her to ask if she'd be joining me in doing another marathon, she told me the devastating news: she had lung cancer. Again the room spun around me: I couldn't believe this was happening again. She'd never smoked, and had led an unusually healthy life. This was a woman who'd done both a BA degree and her first marathon in her 50s, had started doing triathlons in her 60s, and had been contemplating running the entire length of the Thames Path (a distance of 184 miles, or just under 300 kilometres) as a way of 'doing something a bit different' after turning 70. This was a woman who dreamed of being 'a silly grandma aged 90'. Just five months later, we were following her woven-willow coffin outside the country church where her daughter Darian had got married.

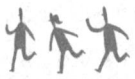

I don't often talk about my mother's death, or that of Aunty Rosie. It's just too painful. But most of the times I've done so have been during marathons, because then I'm doing the very thing that bound us together, the thing that helped me so much in coming to terms with their deaths. As the many signs runners pin to their back in memory of loved ones attest, running really is a sacred, joyous way of remembering the dead. The acclaimed running writer Roger Robinson put it so perfectly when he said: 'Running means more than running. People don't play a round of golf to commemorate a loved one, but they do run races for them.' Knowing that the person we're running in honour of would be proud of the effort we're putting in makes the achievement so much more meaningful. And being able to share our love for a loved one with hundreds or even thousands of other people in a race is a way to keep their memory burning bright.

Sometimes fellow runners have shared a story of loss of their own, which has reminded me that I'm not alone in my grief. A runner called Lauren Goldsmith, for one, told me that she'd run the Greater Manchester Marathon as a way of memorialising her former manager Mike, who sadly died of bowel cancer. 'Mike taught me to never give up and that's exactly what a marathon teaches you, too,' she said. During the Rome Marathon a young woman told me how, as a middle child, her older sister was killed in a car accident and then her younger sister died of pneumonia – all in the space of two years. She'd used running to help her work through her grief. Another runner told me how running had helped her heal after a painful divorce, and how she'd met her current husband, a widower, through running. She told me that the day after their wedding they'd gone together to his late wife's grave and left the bridal bouquet there as a way of saying that she would always be remembered. And I once sat and cried in a gazebo in a park in Milton Keynes with a runner called Atinuke Ogundari, whom I'd buddied up with during the Enigma Week at the Knees Marathon. Atinuke told me that her Mum had died needlessly aged just 49 because the hospital she was taken to in Nigeria simply didn't have the oxygen required to resuscitate her. 'Almost 21 years later my siblings and I still find that shocking, and we're still trying to make sense of her loss,' she said. 'Running has given me a sense of purpose to keep going and live my life as happily as I can because I know my Mum wouldn't want me to be miserable and grieve for ever.' And then there's Yasushi Kokubu, a 70-year-old from Japan, who runs marathons dressed in a pink kimono with a baby gorilla stuffed toy strapped to his back. A friend of his told me that Yasushi never had children and lost his wife several years ago. He views the baby gorilla as the child he and his wife never had and takes it along as he travels the world doing what he loves. So far I've been hugged by Yasushi in marathons in Jerusalem, London and Istanbul, and I hope I'll bump into him in many more to come.

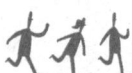

What running taught me about death is that running is the best grief counsellor there is. And that each step can be a tribute to those we love and miss. I feel closest to both my mother and my aunt when I'm running – doing the thing they both loved so much. And when I enter the 'death zone' in a marathon – that long, agonising stretch between halfway and the 20-mile mark that always seems interminable – I can almost feel my mother's hand on my shoulder gently pushing me forwards, and imagine my aunt tripping along beside me keeping my spirits up. When I remember my mother and aunt I like to think of them being together, having a natter. And now, as I run all the marathons my Mum and Aunty Rosie will never get to hear about, I know one thing for sure: whenever I cross a finish line, anywhere in the world, they'll always be there with me, holding my hands aloft.

'Running is an act of remembrance'

'My beloved husband Barry still waits for me at the finish line'

I started running aged 37 to lose weight and since then I've done over 350 races, everything from challenge runs to cross country to 20 marathons. What I'm most proud of is that I've finished every race I've ever started – even when I've had to walk. My ambitions are to run the London Marathon when I'm 70 as well as the New York City and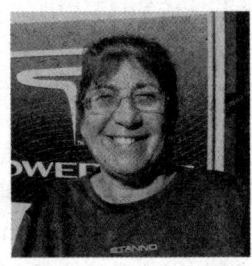
Boston Marathons. I'd still like to be doing 10Ks when I'm 80.

My husband Barry was my greatest supporter – in the 32 years and 18 days we were married he accompanied me to every race and looked after our two children while I ran. 'Get them legs going!' he used to shout from the sidelines. When he died of a stroke aged 58 I couldn't believe it – I felt totally numb. But I ran the Amsterdam half marathon the following month as I knew he'd have wanted me to.

Running helped me cope with my grief by giving me something to focus on. I've seen other widows lose hope, but there's no need to feel lonely, just get out there and join a running club. It's cheap and you'll make loads of friends. I often talk to my husband when I'm out training. I say: 'Where shall we go today, Barry?' I know he's always watching over me, giving me a kick up the backside when I need it and waiting for me at the finish line.

Antoinette 'Aunty' Rendle, 67, Peterborough, England

'I ran a 10K for my Mum when she had only weeks to live'

When I run I think of my Mum. I know she's looking down on me thinking: 'Good for you, Darry, get out there and get running.' All my life my Mum encouraged me to be sporty and she led by example: when I was in my teens she started running and eventually did eight marathons with my cousin Lisa.

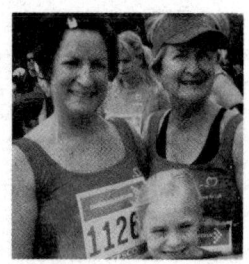

Those times when I was a moody teenager or in my 20s doing my own thing and we came together to jog round the block or run 10K races, those times united us. When she was marathon training and we ran round and round and round the disused airfield near her home we chatted and laughed so much. I cherish those times.

When I was recovering from breast cancer my Mum joined me and my friends at a Race for Life. She ran and walked with my six-year-old daughter Freya so I could run the whole distance. It was only 5K but to me it was an incredible achievement. To have my Mum there, smiling all the way, celebrating my health through our running exploits was magical.

And then there was the 10K that I ran on the hottest day of the year. The 10K I should've been running with my Mum but couldn't because she had only weeks to live. I hated and loved that run. I did it for us, to make her proud, because we had planned to do it, because that's what we did. I could hardly run; I felt drained and the race was a disaster. But I did it. Months later I entered another 10K; this time I did it properly, and although the raw emotions remained it cleared my head as I knew my Mum was encouraging me all the way. Now I don't run a lot, just a bit, but when I run, I think of Mum.

Darian Jeffs, 45, Oakley, England

'My Polish family who were imprisoned in Nazi work camps inspire me to run'

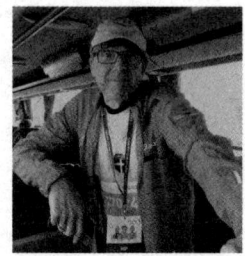

My father came to Sweden as a refugee from Poland in 1948 and during the 375 marathons and ultras I've run I've often thought of the ordeals his family suffered in the Second World War. Whenever I've considered quitting or felt tired during a race I've thought of how they kept going, day after day, even though they were imprisoned in Nazi work camps and had no chance of escape. I know that I enter races of my own free will and that a medal always awaits me at the finish, whereas my Polish family never had any choice about being in the camps and never knew what fate awaited them. Every time I visit Warsaw I place a flower on the Tomb of the Unknown Soldier in their memory.

I often speak to my Dad, who's now turning 90, in my head when I'm struggling in a race and ask him to give me courage. I also talk to my late uncle Joseph, whom, I'm told, I'm the spitting image of. My Dad and Joseph had to exhibit a special kind of endurance as the Iron Curtain prevented them seeing each other for 67 years. Joseph passed away two years after they met up. Sadly, my grandparents never got to know their children had been reunited.

My goal is to run at least 50 marathons in Poland (I'm currently up to 45) as I sense a very special bond with the Polish people. I'm so proud of my Polish heritage that at the age of 45 I had a flag that's half Polish, half Swedish tattooed onto my ankle. Poland rebuilt itself from what were just smouldering ashes after the war. It has a kind of kick-ass mentality – a stamina and a stubbornness – that I recognise in myself as a person and as a runner. I feel that I carry its glorious history in my genes.

Jan Paraniak, 64, Stockholm, Sweden

'I run in honour of my brother who was murdered by a Mexican drug gang'

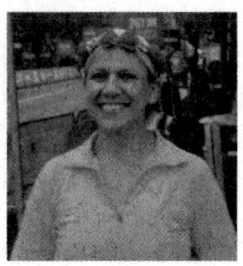

I started running because I got lonely when my husband Victor was away for six months on one of his many deployments with the US Navy. I would run to keep myself sane while taking care of our three kids. I continued to run even when Victor came back from sea as I found it almost meditative. I never imagined running more than 5K until one dreadful day five years ago when my brother Virgilio went missing in Chihuahua, Mexico, where he worked as a cop. When they found him it was too late: he'd been tortured for three days and then killed and dumped on the street like a piece of trash. We think it was just a case of him knowing too much. That day felt like the end of the world. My brother was my best friend and now that he was dead, I felt like dying right then and there. I remember thinking that I'd never get the chance to hug him and tell him how much I loved him, even though he knew that because we'd talked just two days before he disappeared.

I was living in Japan at the time and Victor was on duty aboard ship so I was alone with my children when I heard the news. I didn't have any family I could contact for support, but my kids immediately rang my friend Elsie who dropped everything to come over at 2am and didn't leave my side till 8am when Victor got home.

The next day I got on a plane with my son and flew to Chihuahua to say my last goodbyes to my brother, whom we all called *Nene* ('baby' in Spanish). As I bade him farewell I promised never to think of that terrible day when they found his body but instead vowed I'd only reflect on all the beautiful moments in his life. I didn't want to waste even one minute of my life thinking about horrible people. As a form of therapy I began running barefoot sometimes. It gave me a different sense of running and I thought of my brother's pain while doing it. If he was able to go through three days of being hurt and tortured then I could definitely run a few miles with no shoes on.

Nene was a real 'people person' who often helped others even if he didn't know them, so I decided to honour his memory by doing the same. Things such as buying blankets, shoes and food for the homeless. But I wanted to find another way to pay tribute to him so in 2010 I ran the San Diego Rock 'n' Roll Half Marathon with Victor by my side. Afterwards, I was so inspired by all the comments I got on my Facebook page that I sought an even bigger challenge and entered us into the Verona Marathon. I'm blessed to have a loving and supportive husband who goes along with my craziness – even when I only give him a month's notice to train. By this stage my friend Elsie had been battling breast cancer for 21 months, so I dedicated that race to her and my late brother. I wore the brightest, pinkest compression socks in her honour – they were truly dazzling!

Verona was my first full marathon and I can honestly say that I never had a moment's doubt that I could do it because I knew Nene would be there with me in spirit and cheer me on the whole way. I found the race really tough and Victor tore a hamstring, but we finished together, in Verona's ancient amphitheatre, one of the most romantic settings in the world, in the rain, holding hands. Just like Romeo and Juliet. Almost everyone had already gone home, except Lisa and her husband whom we'd met in the loo queue at the start and who wanted to make sure we'd made it. My stubbornness to finish came from the love I feel when thinking of my brother's and my friend Elsie's courage. People often ask me why I run and all I can say is that I run for those who can't – and that I'll always run with a smile on my face for them.

Cecy Montes, 47, Chihuahua, Mexico

'Running taught me how to cope with terminal illness'

I was born in South Africa and trained as a nurse before marrying Herman, an army officer. During all the years he spent running and being a fitness role model to his men, I was also running: I was running the household, a hospital ward and the bathwater for our three children! Then I got the bug too and Herman and I trained 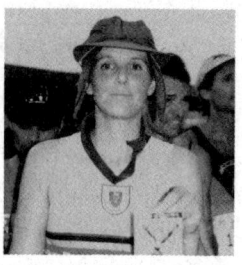 together for countless hours for the Comrades ultramarathon, which I ran twice. At the finish of my first Comrades I was totally exhausted but energised, sore but satisfied, proud but thankful – every emotion rolled into one. After a while, no distance scared me any more, and I did them all, from 10Ks to 100K ultramarathons.

I subsequently moved to Australia and on 2 September 2012 I returned from a two-week stint at an Outback clinic feeling bloated and uncomfortable. Within days it was confirmed that I had mesothelioma: cancer of the intestinal cavity caused by exposure to asbestos. This was akin to being slapped with a death sentence as I was given a month to live unless I had chemotherapy. After two treatments the chemo was stopped because it hadn't relieved the fluid build-up in my belly. After a permanent drain had been inserted I was then told I had four to eight months to live. Strangely, I felt blessed to have been given a time limit for the remainder of my days, an estimate of the time I had left to do what remained to be done. Having had to face cut-off times in races taught me that everything, including life, has a time limit; we've all been given the same amount of time in a day and it's up to each of us to accomplish within it as much as we can. Running taught me a lot that helped me cope with my illness. On many runs I'd battled with the heat or the pain and I constantly reminded myself that I'd been through worse than this before. Running taught me that I had to grit my teeth and push on.

Halfway through my allotted time I got potentially life-threatening peritonitis (infection of the intestines) but what it did, quite miraculously, was stop the fluid accumulating. This allowed me to work a few shifts as a midwife, continue attending kickboxing classes and even enjoy a ride with Herman on our motorbike. By now running was a thing of the past for Herman and me, but we still went for long walks whenever we could.

My Mum and daughters flew out to Australia to be with me at the end. But God had other ideas and all their visas expired before I did. So they all went home again. Then we planned a visit to Israel (where we met Lisa) and the UK for December 2013/January 2014. On our way to England I took a turn for the worse and landed up in hospital, where the exponential growth of my tumours was confirmed. I was now practically bedridden and Herman and I spent many hours reminiscing about our life together. We remembered sharing an energy bar with an exhausted woman sitting, head bowed, at the side of the road, only to have her sprint past us a few minutes later never to be seen again. And we spoke of how we loved people coming up to us after races to thank us for motivating them to finish.

And as for the element of discomfort during these events, I always thanked God that it was my choice to accept these challenges, and that they'd enabled me to have such satisfying experiences with the man I loved as well as my children, either by running shorter races with them or having them cheer me across the finish line with a proud look of 'This is *my* Mom' on their faces.

Colleen van Onselen, 54, Perth, Australia

Colleen crossed the final finish line when she passed away, aged 54, only a few days after dictating this story. Apart from their beautiful almost 36 years together on the road of life, her husband Herman is thankful for the many hours they spent on the road covering the thousands of kilometres they ran in training. Colleen lived life until there was no more life left in her.

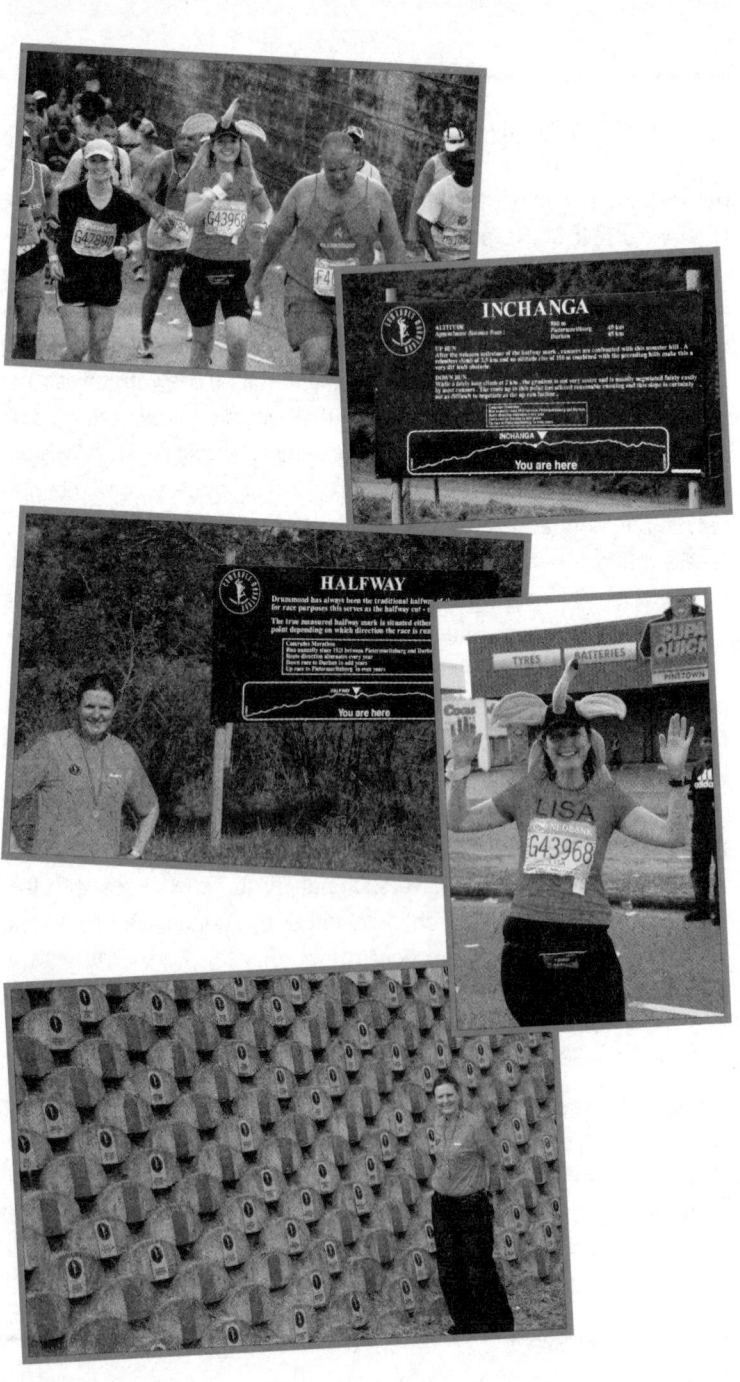

Chapter 7

What running taught me about... dreaming big

As I stood waiting for the start gun of the Comrades Marathon in Pietermaritzburg I squeezed my sister Loren's hand and shed a tear: I couldn't believe we were actually there, two of 12,000 runners, all of whom had made incredible sacrifices or overcome enormous obstacles to be at the start line. Some had struggled to find the R200 (then worth about £15) to pay the entry fee, and had saved up all year to be part of this event. Others had battled injury or risen at 5am every day to fit in the punishing training and still hold down a job. Most of us had run at least 1,000K (over 600 miles) in the preceding six months and all of us had done a marathon in under five hours in order to qualify. I felt honoured to be one of them.

So what brought me to South Africa on 24 May 2009? What drove me to want to run a 91K (56.5-mile) race dubbed 'the world's toughest ultramarathon', which entails doing two marathons one after the other, plus a cheeky 7K (4.4 miles) at the end for good measure? This is a race with a medal no bigger than a 10p coin, and for the majority of runners, who finish between 11 hours and the 12-hour cut-off, it is the pinkish colour of luncheon meat. Waiting for the race to start I had plenty of time to reflect on a journey that had started decades before.

Once a year my father would switch on the TV early in the morning and for one incredible day my family and I would periodically wander into the darkened living room to watch a blond floppy-haired university student called Bruce Fordyce running as if he were a bit late for lectures. 'Brucie', as we fondly called him, would go on to win the Comrades an incredible nine times, and in so doing become a household name. Then, several hours later, we'd reconvene to watch an even more dramatic sight – the final gun. As the clock ticked relentlessly towards the then 11-hour cut-off (an extra hour was added in the year 2000), the entire nation would be glued to their TV sets to see who would make it in time. The finish would be staged with all the drama of a matador delivering the deathblow in a bullfight. After 10 hours and 59 minutes a sombre-suited official would stride to the finish and turn his back on the runners, his eyes on the clock. Beating frantically on the metal advertising hoardings lining the final 200 metres, the crowds would become almost hysterical screaming 'Go! Go! Runnnn! Runnnn!' as the runners desperately attempted to cross the line before the final gun went off. Some would hobble, some would crawl, some would fall down mere metres from the line only to be dragged onto their feet again and be frogmarched to the finish by their fellow runners. And then the official would raise his gun and the crowd would metronomically chant the final ten-second countdown. It seemed as if the entire nation, by the sheer power of collective positive thinking, could will the imperilled stragglers to reach the finish before the gun. 'Bang!' A dozen marshals would sprint across the line, linking arms to form a barrier that no runner could cross. Everyone who didn't finish before that final gun would go home with nothing to show for having run 91K. Not a time. Not a medal. Nothing. No matter if they missed the gun by even a single second.

I witnessed this intriguing spectacle throughout my childhood, and heard many tales about the race from my sister, who'd run it three times in her 20s. I secretly envied the runners I saw on that TV screen every year. Secretly, because I loathed anything to do with athletics; I'd been humiliated one too many times on sports day when they'd often be making the presentations on the podium before I'd even crossed the finish line.

Then, three years and six marathons after I'd started running, I began contemplating doing the Comrades Marathon. By then I'd realised that this was one race I simply had to do if I'd ever be taken seriously as a runner in my home country of South Africa. When I'd told schoolfriends back home about my metamorphosis into a marathon runner they'd initially been astonished ('No!? Really? You?'), as I think I'd been unofficially voted The Girl Least Likely To Succeed At Anything Athletic, but then almost immediately this had been followed by: 'So are you going to do Comrades?' Because in South Africa it's not enough to do a marathon, you need to have run this iconic race to have any street cred at all in the running community. London? New York? Pah! Those are just *qualifiers* for Comrades.

But my Comrades dream, like a mirage, kept receding. Whenever I snuck a look at the scary six-month training programme my heart would sink and I'd put it off for yet another year. I even stuck a photocopy of the course's elevation profile in my study, but made sure it was inside a cupboard because every time I looked at it I felt faint. Ironically, writing *Running Made Easy* also got in the way of my dream as lack of time meant I had the perfect excuse not to train.

Eventually, aged 40, having recently celebrated ten years of being a runner, my Canadian friend Bridget and I started talking seriously about Comrades. Via email and Skype we endlessly analysed how we were going to do it. Most crucially, we'd have to get faster in order to achieve the sub-five-hour qualifying time. A whole lot faster. My PB for a marathon was 5h19, and my average time for that distance was 5h45. Worse still, I needed to cut virtually an hour from my last marathon time – could that actually be done? I didn't have a clue. The thought of doing the training petrified me as there were weekends, for example, when you were expected to run 30K (18.6 miles) on a Saturday, and the same again the next day!

Then, in November 2008, Bridget sent me an email informing me that she'd entered Comrades and detailing all the training she'd done for the past six weeks in preparation for her Comrades qualifier. I was appalled. She was running 5K to 8K (3 to 5 miles) five days a week, and on the sixth she was already doing a half marathon. She was deadly serious about this Comrades thing and I had a simple choice to make: was I going to walk/run the walk/run with her, or just continue talking the talk? That very day I went for a 'test' 10K run with my husband to assess my current speed and was horrified when my stopwatch recorded a time of 78 minutes. To have even a sniff at qualifying I had to be able to do 10K (6.2 miles) in, at most, 71 minutes.

'I'll never do it. I just can't run any faster,' I despondently declared, mentally throwing in the towel there and then.

Looking me straight in the eye, knowing full well how much this ambition meant to me, Graham said quietly but with great conviction: 'Lisa, this is only the beginning – now you know where you stand. You had to start somewhere.'

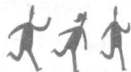

I went home feeling defeated and for the rest of the afternoon wrestled with the dilemma of whether or not to enter. This was the dream I'd hardly dared dream. I really, really, really wanted to do it, even though I knew the idea was as improbable and unlikely as teaching a hippo to hip-hop. I'd read that the average age of first-time Comrades finishers was 41, so it was the perfect year for me to do it. And I also knew that the only thing that would be different the following year would be being a year older. So I emailed Bridget to let her know I'd be joining her, went online and entered, and the very next day did a 21K (13-mile) training run.

It was hell. As I ran through London's dark and dirty streets that cold winter's evening the only thought that kept crossing my mind was 'Why? Why exactly do I want to run Comrades?' I knew that I had to find a better reason than to astonish my schoolfriends. I knew that just reaching the start line was going to require me to dig very deep into reserves of courage and perseverance I wasn't sure I possessed. After many miles of soul-searching I stumbled across my motivation: I would run in celebration of my beloved Mum. The moment I made that decision I believed I'd finish, though I also knew I'd be assailed by an army of doubts along the way.

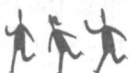

The weeks of training through one of the UK's bitterest winters soon became months. I had ditched my original too-tough-ain't-tough-enough training schedule and was now following a far more doable one devised by former Comrades coach Don Oliver (a veteran of 19 Comrades). It had been sent to me by Nikki Campbell, the South African founder of Also Ran Runners, a website for Comrades wannabes. Nikki's help, all given free of charge, was invaluable. She became my mentor, advising me on everything from time management ('Don't waste time doing unnecessary things such as leg rubs, stopping to chat to friends') to toilet stops ('Don't queue for toilets: there's plenty of vegetation en route').

The programme involved having one rest day and running between 5K (3.1 miles) and 10K (6.2 miles) on five days of the week, with a long run ranging from 20K (12.4 miles) to 65K (40.4 miles) at the weekend. Even this programme looked extremely intimidating at first, but I told myself to just focus on what was required each day. I knew that that 65K run was lurking in the future, but I tried to ignore it and just keep reminding myself of how amazing I'd feel once I could call myself a Comrades runner. I knew I'd come a long way since starting running ten years ago – and fervently hoped I'd be able to go further still.

Every day I would bargain with myself about when I'd go out for my run. I work from home so I had the entire day at my disposal, yet several times I had to go running at 10pm because I'd procrastinated for so long. Each Sunday I'd have the same great debate with myself – whether or not to go for my long run. I usually ended up going out eventually (the times I bailed on my training, I felt unbelievably guilty all week), but not before I'd exhausted every possible reason and excuse not to. And each time I had my post-workout shower I'd write the word 'COMRADES' in the condensation inside the shower door as a way of keeping my dream alive.

My husband started accompanying me on my Sunday runs just to get me out of the door before my agonised moping drove him mad. Graham's a much faster runner than me and spent a lot of the time running backwards! Whenever I lagged behind he'd turn round, point to the empty space beside him and say: 'I want you *here*!' He also enjoyed tormenting me with a game we called 'I declare a hill'. I'd decided that my race strategy for Comrades would be to walk all the uphills and run the downhill and flat sections, so I wanted to practise that in training. Graham had other ideas. The minute I called out 'I declare a hill!', meaning that I'd spotted an incline and wanted to walk up it, he'd rush back to my side and annoyingly encourage me to sprint instead.

'The only way to get faster is to run faster,' he'd endlessly intone. I would've strangled him if I could have caught up with him. And when we got home we'd writhe around on the rug in front of the telly doing our stretches, mugs of steaming hot tea to hand, moaning like mad about how hard it had all been.

But not everyone had as much faith in me as Graham. One day I was asked by another runner what I was training for. 'Believe it or not, Comrades,' I replied. Hearing that, the runner simply snorted and ran off. Being one of the slowest runners I know, I could well understand his reaction. But it devastated me nonetheless, and when I got home I sobbed for over an hour, feeling a horrible mix of shame and embarrassment. The little evil monkey inside my head just wouldn't stop chattering: 'Yes, what makes you think *you* can do Comrades? You're the unathletic one. The slow one. You're not even a runner, you're a jogger and a joke.' And so it went on, and on. I fervently wished I'd kept my dream secret so that no one would be able to say 'I told you so' when I failed.

This funk lasted for a few days and had a catastrophic effect on my training: I stopped running. My dream was evaporating like the soft edges of a cloud on a summer's day. And then it hit me. I was a hypnotherapist, for Pete's sake: I knew precisely what to do to hurdle a confidence crisis. I'd taught it to dozens of my clients, and yet I wasn't applying it to myself. That evening I sat down in front of my computer and started watching YouTube footage of the runners who crossed the finish line in my predicted time of just under 12 hours. Unlike the footage I'd seen as a child, these runners weren't crawling or zigzagging deliriously across it. No, they were finishing strongly, with smiles a mile wide. And many of them were in their sixties and seventies for crying out loud. I sat in front of the screen for several hours reviewing the clips, imagining what it would be like to run around the stadium with the crowds going crazy in the stands. I allowed myself to feel the sense of achievement, the euphoria. Tears streamed down my face. I got goosebumps.

Now I knew what my training plan had meant when it said 'Running Comrades is 80 per cent mental.' It was. I had mental strength; I'd inherited it from my mother, in spades. From then on, I did self-hypnosis every night before falling asleep, repeatedly visualising making my Mum proud by crossing that finish line. I just *knew* my self-belief would see me through.

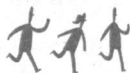

My courage and confidence restored, I started running again, and began attending speed-training sessions at my running club. I also did endless squats, lunges and leg-strengthening work, such as sitting in an imaginary chair, proudly working up, over time, from just ten seconds to a full three minutes. I also religiously followed the moderate-carb, higher-protein, veg-crammed eating plan that I later wrote a book about *(Adore Yourself Slim)*. And then, on 2 February 2009, London was hit by the heaviest snowfall in 18 years and came to a grinding halt. So did my training. The pavements had turned into ice rinks and for days I was trapped indoors. Frantic that I wouldn't be ready for my qualifying marathon in Seville later that month I decided to risk skidding my way up to our high street where I hoped the council would have cleared away some of the snow. Sure enough, I found a 200-metre long stretch of pavement that was mostly free of ice and snow and began running back and forth along it. I was actually quite enjoying myself when, about halfway through the 80 laps I had to do, I became aware of a group of hoody-wearing teenagers congregated outside a pizza shop. A family friend had been viciously attacked by a drug addict at a takeaway on the very same road, so I eyed them nervously each time I ran past. After a few more laps it became obvious that they'd noticed me as they kept shooting glances in my direction, and then I started to suspect they were talking about me.

'Right, that's it, I'm heading home,' I thought fearfully. 'There's no way I'm going to have my head kicked in for the sake of a run.' The entire group turned to watch me as I ran past them for the last time, my heart pounding even more than normal, desperate to get back to the safety of my home. One of them called out to me, and at first I couldn't quite believe what I'd just heard.

'Keep going, lady,' he shouted. 'You're a LEGEND!'

My grimace turned into a grin, and with a huge double thumbs-up I made the decision to keep going for the remaining 40 laps. I even started looking forward to the supportive smiles and nods I got from my hoody-boy cheerleaders every time I passed.

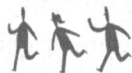

When the time came to run my qualifying marathon with my sister in Seville, I stuck religiously to my prearranged pacing schedule through the orange-tree-lined streets, despite having somehow forgotten the list of splits I'd typed out for myself and regardless of the fact that my GPS watch mysteriously refused to register distance on the day, only time. I relentlessly focused on doing 6.7 minutes per kilometre and didn't chat to a soul, which for once wasn't a major challenge as so few of the other runners spoke English. Only afterwards did Loren mention that she thought my time-keeping was a bit dubious because, as she put it, 'I think you were doing Monkey Maths: what on earth is point seven of a minute?' I still can't tell you how it all worked, but it did. I became so emotional while running the final 400 metres inside the Olympic stadium that I almost couldn't continue as my wracking sobs were affecting my breathing. However, I managed to sprint the final 200 metres and beat every other runner ahead of me. I'd qualified. My time of 4h39 meant I'd just run a marathon 40 minutes faster than I ever had before. When I got home, Graham had painted a huge banner and strung it across our dining room: 'QUEEN OF THE HILL 4:39' it proclaimed in honour of all the hill training we'd done together in preparation. 'Declaring' hills had worked – I was stronger and faster than I'd ever been.

With the qualifying marathon out of the way, the next hurdle was doing an ultramarathon in training – something I'd never attempted before. Don Oliver's programme advised doing three distances ranging from 50K (31 miles) to 65K (40.4 miles) in April and May to get us used to spending large amounts of time on our feet. Many South African runners choose to run the 56K (34.8-mile) Two Oceans Marathon in Cape Town, which has a cut-off of seven hours, as one of the three, so I decided to stage my own solo event in London and run it on the same day. On Easter Saturday I planned to run northwards from my home in Croydon across the Thames to Hampstead Heath and back. I felt unbelievably nauseous when I woke up (probably the result of spending the night in a state of fear at what I was proposing to do) and only got going by 11.30am. On reaching Camden Market after 21K (13 miles) I was unexpectedly joined by a man who was wandering around holding an Alan Shearer doll. He was asking female passers-by,

'Do you want to be a footballer's wife?' He claimed to have recently been released from prison (I didn't dare ask why he'd been jailed) but was amazingly good company for the hour he chose to run with me. I reached home with four minutes to spare, right on target, having left my new friend and his doll on Hampstead Heath. Having run/walked further than I'd ever dreamed possible, I was utterly elated – at long last Comrades was within my grasp.

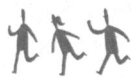

And then I experienced my first setback – Bridget had injured herself during her qualifying marathon and wouldn't be doing Comrades. (Fortunately my sister Loren had also agreed to do it with me, so I knew I wouldn't be lining up at the start line alone.) This was swiftly followed by setback number two, a hamstring injury. A few days after my 56K run I had an ache in the back of my left thigh that got progressively more painful and was eventually diagnosed as a hamstring tear. I was terrified of making it worse, but even more petrified of being undertrained, and turned to my physiotherapist Leslie Watson, who'd won the 55-mile London to Brighton ultramarathon twice, for advice.

'If you tell me not to run Comrades with this injury, I won't,' I told her as she massaged my injured thigh.

'Not run Comrades?' she replied, with her trademark Scottish lilt. 'If you said you wanted to *win* it, I'd say "Perhaps not this year." But *run* it? Basically it's just a fast walk.'

Well, that settled it. I had the medical all-clear. Darn!

My schedule dictated that I had to do two more ultramarathons before C-Day, but when the day of my longest scheduled run, a

65K epic, dawned, I followed the advice Leslie had given me and ran for just 30K. Thank goodness I did, as the caffeinated gels I was trialling for the first time gave me a terrible stitch and made me burp continuously as I shuffled my way through the gritty streets of Catford. I later learned you're not supposed to take them neat but with plenty of water. The third ultra never materialised either as my hamstring was just too painful. Truth to tell, I was thrilled that I had a cast-iron reason for not doing it as all those ultralong Sunday runs had become a huge drag. I felt fairly confident that as my qualifier had been much faster than I'd anticipated, I'd have a good shot at finishing.

Having flown to South Africa a few days previously, and having had an emergency session of physio on my hamstring that morning, we drove up from Durban to the Comrades start line in Pietermaritzburg the day before the race. I hardly dared look out of the window in case it revealed too much about the daunting task that lay ahead. Instead, I spent my time reading the good luck cards I'd been sent, along with my mentor Nikki's most-inspiring emails: 'You are going to love Comrades,' she'd written. 'It's a journey more than a race. Don't fret about it, be excited that you are brave enough to accept the challenge. Then just go out and enjoy the day, knowing that the spectators on the side of the road are secretly wishing they were you. The most important thing on the day is to BELIEVE IN YOURSELF.'

The night before Comrades there was a good omen. We had dinner at Pesto, an Italian restaurant that was so packed with pasta-seeking runners that we had to sit at a table hastily set up for us in the car park. But this was no ordinary table. It had the best imaginable view: that of Brucie, the Comrades Legend himself, now 53, who was also running the next day, eating his pasta at an outdoor gazebo.

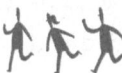

Race day. After months of physiotherapy, sports massage, personal-training sessions and £200 worth of supplements plus £40 for the fetching flamingo hat with flappable wings I'd specially imported from America, Loren and I were finally on the start line in front of Pietermaritzburg City Hall. I felt like a warrior squaring up to face a formidable array of enemies: the heat, the hills (towering monsters known as the Big Five), the road and, most scary of all, the clock.

Just before 5.30am we sang the South African national anthem and the Zulu folksong 'Shozaloza', which means 'Go forward, make way for the next man'. I felt so very proud to be South African that day. Next up was the goosebump-inducing sound of 'Chariots of Fire', and then we heard the long-awaited crowing of a cock, a recording of Comrades regular Max Trimborn, who started this unique tradition in 1948 when he gave an ear-piercing imitation of an awakening cockerel just before the start, something he continued to do until his death 32 years later.

When the gun went off we surged forward through the sleeping streets of Pietermaritzburg, nodding to silently acknowledge the clapping of the townsfolk, many of whom had come to spectate in their pyjamas. As we headed down Polly Shortts, the first hill, one of the Zulu runners cried: 'Eaaaasy!

Eaaaaassssy does it! Speed kills!' We smiled in recognition at the wisdom of these words – running lore has it that running too fast early on can cost you dearly in the second half. Then he was at it again: 'You must talk now, because you won't be able to once you reach Pinetown!' At this the veterans laughed and started to talk, but we novices shuddered at the thought of what lay ahead and remained silent.

It wasn't long before my feet started to hurt. In a last-ditch attempt to gain any possible advantage I'd taken a friend's advice and thereby made a fundamental error: I'd donned not only two pairs of running socks but also a pair of flight socks. I'd never run in this combo before, and the unexpected volume of material in my shoes was squishing my toes tightly together, which swiftly resulted in some very uncomfortable blisters – with 80K (50 miles) left to run. Nonetheless, I faithfully tried to follow the splits Nikki had sent me that I'd printed out on a paper bracelet protected from my sweat by sticky tape. I was wearing both my Garmin and a stopwatch as the former only had a battery life of ten hours and I was anticipating finishing in 11h45. I have incredibly scrawny wrists, and my Garmin had bruised me terribly in Seville, so I wore a fetching piece of bright orange bubble wrap under it.

As planned, Loren and I conserved energy by walking up the hills and running the downhills and flats. Every time we slowed to a walk I reminded myself of the mantras in my Comrades training programme: 'Walk with pride and purpose. And never, never, never bail.' At about the 20K (12.4-mile) mark my sister said she couldn't keep up the pace and so I very reluctantly left her (she later failed to meet the final cut-off and so had to catch a bail bus to the finish).

When I'd told my Dad that I was going to attempt Comrades he had two pieces of advice: 'Don't run in fancy dress; this is a serious race, not some kind of carnival. And whatever you do, don't talk, save your breath for running.' Of course I wasn't about to listen to him on the first one, but I conceded he might have a point with the second. Which is why, despite being a champion chat-runner, I vowed to remain silent throughout the race. There was just one impediment, however: South Africans are incredibly friendly and the race ethos actively encourages runners to get to know each other en route. This is because, although the name Comrades is derived from the First World War veterans it was created to commemorate, it's also come to signify something rather mystical called 'the Comrades spirit'. To foster this camaraderie (or should that be Comraderie?) runners are issued with a second colour-coded race number, to be worn on their back, which discloses not only their name, age and nationality but also their running CV: how many times they've finished Comrades; whether they're going for a back-to-back medal which is awarded to those who do Comrades twice in successive years; and whether they're going for the almost unimaginable Green Number that's awarded to those who finish ten Comrades. With the help of this simple but inspired icebreaker every single runner is on first-name terms with the whole field. Which is why I was constantly being wished good luck for my first race, asked how I was doing and, rather amazingly, being told over and over again whenever I mentioned my blisters or hapless hamstring,

'Well, the most important thing is just that you *enjoy* the race.' Nearing the halfway mark, I thought they were all as crazy as a soup sandwich. '*Enjoy* the race?' What in heaven's name was enjoyable about silently slogging up seemingly interminable hills with throbbing feet and an aching hamstring while casting anxious glances at my Garmin?

'This race is terribly overrated!' I recall thinking grimly. I was shocked by the enormity of that thought. That this dream I'd had since I was a girl just wasn't all it was cracked up to be. Truth be told, I was *bored*.

And then I bumped into my Comrades mentor Nikki, who told me I was looking good and what a great run she was having. 'Every year I ask myself the same question: do I want to be anywhere else in the whole world except here on this day?' she said. 'And the answer, of course, is always no.'

I didn't reply (Dad's orders) but mentally I was moodily muttering, 'Yes, Nikki, as a matter of fact I can think of about a thousand places I'd rather be right now – even sitting in a traffic jam would be more fun.'

Nikki ran on and my agonising trudge continued. By halfway I seriously considered giving up as I was 25 minutes behind schedule and thought it would make sense to spare myself the pain of running for another six hours only to go home without a medal. But then I remembered something Nikki had written in one of her emails: 'I've found that I catch up later during the run... it's not all over if you fall behind on Don's chart.' Then I recalled the runner who'd snorted in disbelief when he'd heard what I proposed to do and my resolve stiffened: 'I'll show him,' I thought. 'I'm not going to give him the satisfaction of knowing I pulled out before I was forced out.'

And then, when I needed it most, I met a wonderful runner whose excitement at running Comrades for the first time was infectious. I wasn't intending to talk to Barbara and only wanted to ask her which country she was from, having noticed from a distance that her race number had a blue background denoting she was a foreigner. I also noticed her blonde ponytail swinging from side to side as she gaily chatted to the runner next to her. 'She looks happy,' I remember thinking, 'and I'm not.' The minute I heard she was from Canada, like my friend Bridget, I just couldn't help myself: I simply had to break my vow of silence. My Dad's advice was discarded like an empty water bottle and from then on we chatted as if we were the good friends we later became. No longer bored or lonely, and with someone who wholeheartedly embraced my 'I declare a hill' philosophy, the kilometres flew by. We didn't even break step (or draw breath) at the feared downhill sections at Fields Hill and Cowies Hill, where grown men, having run a punishing 65K by that point, were rumoured to cry as they clung to the crash barriers, their quads screeching in pain.

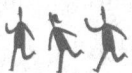

With 21K to go Barbara turned to me and said, 'I think we've made it! We've got a whole four hours to do a half marathon and even if we crawl from here, we'll finish!'

My heart soared but I wasn't going to count any chickens, and insisted we keep up our run/walk strategy all the way to the finish. Having seen the sea at Durban glinting in the distance for what seemed like an eternity, the next thing we knew we were running through the centre of town towards the Sahara Stadium Kingsmead. The spectators lining the streets were cheering wildly, delighted that we'd made it, willing us on, clapping or punching their fists into the air. Making eye contact with as many spectators as I could it was almost as if I was crowd surfing, with each supporter passing me along to their neighbour for the next dose of encouragement.

We entered the stadium and I caught the scent of crushed grass underfoot and heard a deafening roar. All of a sudden I saw Graham in the stands, and he handed me the huge poster I'd made in honour of my Mum. It read: 'Running in celebration of Leoné Jackson. Mom. Wife. Christian. Marathon Runner. Inspiration.' I held it up as I crossed the finish line I'd crossed hundreds of times in my dreams. I'd finished Comrades in 11h43, two minutes faster than my target time. The one person I most wanted to share the moment with wasn't there – my Mum. However, I took solace from the fact that she'd been with me every step of the way, both in spirit and in the photo of her I'd pinned to my back. I knew I'd done her proud and that, as I celebrated, somewhere up on high she was cheering like crazy.

So what has running taught me about dreaming big? That's easy: don't snort when someone shares their dream with you. Over the years and over many miles I've felt immensely privileged when runners have divulged their dreams – and the fears that inevitably go hand in hand with them – to me. And, even when their dreams have seemed impossible, improbable and downright crazybonkers (Run seven marathons in seven days on seven continents? Complete 300 marathons? Circumnavigate Iceland on foot? Run 250 miles in one go?), I've remembered the single snort that so nearly derailed my Comrades and have instead responded with enthusiasm and encouragement. I've made it my mission to be a cheerleader rather than a doubter. I want those I meet to remember me with the same warm and fuzzy fondness I experience when I think of Graham, Leslie, Nikki, Don and Barbara. One of the nicest things anyone's ever said to me was when I returned to the UK after Comrades and told the snorting story to two close friends, Lize and Paulo. 'He really did that?' they gasped, outraged on my behalf. 'We *always* knew you'd make it. That guy? He just doesn't *know* you like we do.' I was incredibly touched by the faith they'd had in me because, in all honesty, I hadn't actually known whether I'd make it or not. And it was only the amazingly positive people I surrounded myself with, the people who continually topped up my tank of courage, who got me through.

Not snorting aside, running has also taught me that nothing is impossible, and that the task ahead of you is never greater than the strength within you. If you have a dream, and it's truly something you want, you will find a way to make it happen. My current dream is to join the 100 Marathon Club, hopefully around the time this book is published. It's been tough finding the time to run a marathon virtually every fortnight while holding down a job and writing this book. It's been an even greater challenge finding marathons that have cut-offs generous enough to allow me to finish! But I'm doing it. And when I'm presented with my blue-and-yellow 100 Marathon Club T-shirt there'll be three badges sewn onto it. Two will be the badges I got for running Comrades (yes, I went back the following year and did it again), which are still the biggest dream-come-true moments of my running life. And one will be a NASA badge I bought at the John F. Kennedy Space Center at Cape Canaveral. During our visit to 'America's gateway to the universe' I was moved to tears hearing JFK's 1961 speech to Congress when he dramatically announced the ambitious goal of sending an American to the moon: 'We choose to go to the moon in this decade and do the other things, not because they are easy, but because they are hard.' That speech perfectly summed up why I run marathons and ultramarathons rather than shorter races: it's precisely *because* distance running is so darn hard that it's so darn satisfying. The second reason I'll be sewing a NASA badge onto my T-shirt? Because when I was growing up there were two things most people would've predicted I'd never be: an astronaut and a marathon runner. I'm not an astronaut today, but I'm unbelievably proud that I reached for the stars and became a runner. I'm beyond thrilled that I've lived up to the challenge Ralph Waldo Emerson threw down when he wrote: 'Dare to live the life you have dreamed for yourself. Go forward and make your dreams come true.'

'We dreamt it – and then we did it!'

'It felt incredible running seven marathons in seven days on seven continents'

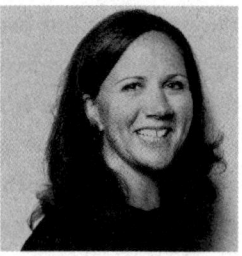

Every time I think back to my 7x7x7 Challenge it always makes me feel humble and a little emotional, as people I'd never met before just turned up and helped me achieve a hugely important goal. When I decided to run seven marathons in seven days on seven continents I contacted running clubs around the world to ask them to help me devise my routes and accompany me when I ran.

I first flew to the Falklands and after that ran marathons in Santiago in Chile, Los Angeles, Sydney, Singapore, Cairo and finally London. I managed to get a whole row of seats to myself for all the flights except LA to Sydney – I'm really tall and for that flight I was crammed into a single economy seat for 14 hours and could barely move.

In the event, I got so much support from local runners that the hardest part wasn't the running itself but ensuring I didn't miss my flight connections. Disaster was narrowly avoided in Cairo when my flight was delayed, but after some frantic negotiations I managed to book myself onto another one. Lisa had jokingly asked if I could run the London leg a little slower so she'd have time to leave work and get to the finish line to greet me. Fortunately, the delay meant I didn't have to run slowly as by then I was so excited I just sprinted like a madwoman past all my colleagues in the City who'd come out to cheer me.

Imagining the finish line had kept me going all week, but seeing my friends and family standing on The Mall waving flags and celebrating the fact I'd run 183.4 miles (295 kilometres) in 35.5 hours was unbelievable. Real life outdid imagination big time. My 7x7x7 taught me two things: that there are some amazing people in this world, and that if you focus all your energy on something you can achieve it.

Marie-Louise Stenild, 38, London, England

'I'm aiming to run 300 marathons'

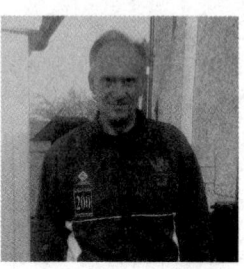

I quit smoking on New Year's Day 1990 and the following year ran the London Marathon. I had to work extremely hard to build up my fitness after smoking 20 to 30 cigarettes a day for 18 years! When the big day arrived I was so nervous that I struggled to move let alone run in the first two miles, but then the crowds inspired me. Running towards Big Ben was the most amazing experience: I had tears in my eyes seeing my family screaming with joy at the finish. That was the moment I knew that this was something I wanted to do as often as possible and that was when I joined the wonderful family of marathon runners. After 221 marathons I still get a big buzz when I complete one; the moment this disappears I'll know it's time to stop.

My next target is to run 300 marathons so that I can be included in the World Megamarathon rankings. Marathon running is an extraordinary experience but it involves a lot of hard work. I've found that a positive attitude to training and competing is the key: respect the distance, respect your fellow competitors and don't allow your race times to affect your enjoyment. People say I've been lucky not to pick up injuries but I think you make your own luck. I listen to my body, avoid punishing speed sessions as they caused injuries in the past, and use a marathon as a training run for the next one. Every marathon provides a clean canvas: sometimes you paint a beautiful picture, sometimes you mess up. The marathon community will support you, encourage you and compete with you until you manage to paint another beautiful picture.

Nick Kyritsis, 60, Croydon, England

I'd wanted to do the 156-mile (251K) Marathon des Sables in the Sahara for ages but as a single mum of two finding the money and time to train were an issue. I bought a money box and ten years later, despite being a plodder and knowing that these challenges are full of 'dark places' mentally, I lined up at the start. The first day was horrendous as carrying a heavy pack while battling the sand and the 50°C heat really sapped me, but breaking each day's distance down into little chunks helped. I'd put my head down and force myself to count 100 steps before I could look up again. I was very proud to finish but truly believe anyone can achieve what I did if they want to enough, as I'm just a normal runner – albeit a stubborn one!

Katharine Redman, 48, Petersfield, England

After crossing the finish line of my first marathon in New York at the age of 35, I knew life would never be the same: running had somehow manifested a drive in me I'd never known existed. Later, aged 38, and having done 21 marathons, I set myself a target of doing 40 marathons before my fortieth birthday. Then I upped that to 100, which I achieved last year, aged 40. My next goal was to complete all six World Marathon Majors (New York City, Berlin, London, Chicago, Tokyo and Boston: runners who've completed all of them get a special certificate, see page 310) in my fortieth year, which I also managed to do. Now I'm aiming to complete a World City A–Z Marathon challenge I invented myself.

For me a marathon isn't measured by time but by the intensity of the running experience and the friendships made along the way. Each marathon has a special significance in my life, a medal engraved as a memory.

So Mei Chan (aka May Chan), 40, London, England

'I dreamt of running 250 miles in one go'

I try to push myself out of my comfort zone at least once a year, so after completing the 145-mile (233.4K) Grand Union Canal Race from Birmingham to London in 2014, I was looking for my next challenge. I found it in the Thames Ring 250, the UK's longest non-stop trail race, which involves running the equivalent of nine-and-a-half back-to-back marathons (i.e. 250 miles, or 402.3 kilometres) in less than 100 hours – with the bare minimum of sleep.

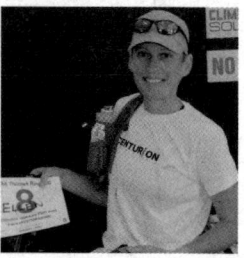

From the minute I signed up for the race I started my planning and read every blog ever written about it. As I knew I wouldn't be able to think clearly at times during the race, I did all my thinking beforehand, filling nine carrier bags with the things I'd need at each checkpoint. I also incorporated four 100-mile (161K) races into my training plan, doing them without a pacer or crew as I knew neither was allowed for this event.

The race started at 10am and, as I'd prepared a race plan, I didn't worry too much when everyone sprinted away from me. The day just seemed to get hotter and hotter so I ran in the sunny sections and took walk breaks in the shady parts. The stretch to the second checkpoint was, strangely, the hardest: I saw lots of runners throwing up along the course and felt very nauseous myself. However, I managed to reach it and made sure I ate everything I'd packed in my bag. I was now way behind schedule but decided I'd rather have a slow finish than a fast DNF (Did Not Finish).

By now it was nightfall. I was so tired that it scared me, but the company of three other runners was a lifesaver as we just kept chatting and moving forward. I spent day two on my own, having parted company with the others, but was rejoined by two of them during the second night.

After 156 miles (251K) I was on my own again but just happy to be past the halfway point. I vaguely remember asking a statue for directions at some stage: at first I thought he was being rude when he didn't reply! Halfway through night three I started feeling really sleepy. The temperature dropped dramatically and there was a thick fog over the Oxford Canal. I was also suffering from constant hallucinations: I kept seeing people and animals up in the trees and floating past me.

About another hour down the trail I blacked out and fell into the canal. I was glad this happened as I was now wide awake and my feet were numb and therefore no longer hurt, plus I had to keep running no matter what or get hypothermia! At around mile 200 (kilometre 322) I realised that I really wasn't cut out for long-distance running: the trail now consisted of shoulder-high wet grass and I found myself crying like a child who'd dropped her ice-cream cone. I was running and crying and mumbling 'I can't stop, I can't stop'. My feet were now on fire. When I got to the next checkpoint I slept for 35 minutes, waking up a whole new woman.

With just under ten miles to go I hit the biggest ultra-high I've ever experienced. I listened to the 1980s song 'Mickey' and began dancing while running, using my water bottle as a pretend microphone. People were looking at me like I was crazy but I didn't care! And then, at long last, I ran around a corner and saw the finish. Everyone cheered, but since it was around midnight and we were in a residential area, they had to do so at a whisper. My watch told me I'd been running for 85 hours and 12 minutes. The end was almost bittersweet: I was so proud to have survived but sad that the amazing adventure was over.

I came sixth out of the 19 finishers — 20 runners dropped out. In total I had two hours' sleep and had gained two small blisters, some serious bragging rights, and a pain in my neck from the massive medal. I know completing this race came down to one thing: self-belief. I never used the words 'if', 'try', or 'attempt', it was always 'I will finish'. We're all capable of so much more than we think. I still remember the days when running a 5K scared me!

Ellen Cottom, 41, Portsmouth, England

'I ran around Iceland after nearly being paralysed'

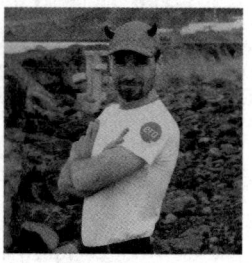

The reason I dreamt a crazy dream of running around Iceland was that I wanted to find a way to celebrate not having to spend the rest of my life in a wheelchair. Five years before, aged 33, I'd nearly been killed in a car accident that shattered one of my vertebrae and my doctors feared I'd never walk again. I'd been a keen runner and had run the Prague Marathon every year for ten years. Six days after the operation, in which four eight-centimetre-long titanium screws were inserted into my spine, I discharged myself from hospital. I couldn't sit, as it was too painful, so I began rebuilding my strength by standing up for short periods. After a month I could stay on my feet for eight hours, and after another few months I tried running again. It was agonising at first as I felt the jolt of every step in my spine, but seven months after the operation I ran the Prague Marathon, crying tears of joy after crossing the cobbled finish line.

A few years later I began to hatch my plan of circumnavigating Iceland to raise funds for disabled sportspeople. Covering the 1,300 kilometres meant running more than a marathon a day for 30 days so I asked my girlfriend Bára if she'd tag along in a camper van to support me. The only hiccup was that by then we'd have our two-month-old in tow. Thankfully, she said yes. (Bára's made of tough stuff: when she was seven months' pregnant we went camping with Lisa and her husband in the Kokorin Woods outside Prague and, like the rest of us, she slept on the bare ground under an overhanging rock.)

Five years to the day after my accident I set off from Reykjavik. For the first ten days the weather was abysmal, with headwinds gusting up to 80 kph, but after that the sun came out allowing me to appreciate the stark but spectacular Icelandic scenery: black-sand beaches, glaciers and still-smoking volcanoes. Despite two near-death experiences (one with a texting motorist, the other with an overtaking bus) I reached Reykjavik where I was given an honour guard by 40 supporters, many of them disabled. Having spent over 163 hours on the road my first thought on finishing was: 'I wish Iceland was bigger!'

Well, barring another volcanic eruption, I realised Iceland wasn't going to get any bigger anytime soon, but I wanted an excuse to return so I decided to traverse Iceland from north to south the following year. This time Bára and our son, Robin, couldn't accompany me so I had to pack everything I'd need into a running stroller. It weighed 50 kg and considerably hampered my progress, especially when I had to ford Iceland's many rivers. By far the worst day was day eight when I was forced to run 90 kilometres to reach the safety of a mountain hut before appalling weather struck. It was exhausting and I was tempted to stop and sleep several times, but I knew that if I did I'd probably die of exposure, so I pushed on into the night, finally reaching the hut at 4am. I had to hole up there for 40 hours waiting for the storm to pass before I could get going again. After that it was plain sailing and, 14 days and 556 kilometres after I set off, I finished my challenge.

Of course, no sooner had I reached the southern shore than I started dreaming up another adventure: this time I decided to run 963 kilometres across Iceland from east to west in three weeks. Again the weather refused to play ball and on day 18 ferocious winds meant I had no option but to take an unscheduled 24-hour rest. The day before I finished I was sitting in an outdoor hot spring with two friends drinking Czech beer and suddenly it dawned on me that I was just about to become the first person in the world to have run around, across and the length of Iceland. Words can't describe how elated I felt. The best bit? Knowing that I'd run to raise funds for those who will never run again. I was delighted that achieving my big dreams meant others would have a chance of achieving theirs.

René Kujan, 41, Prague, Czech Republic

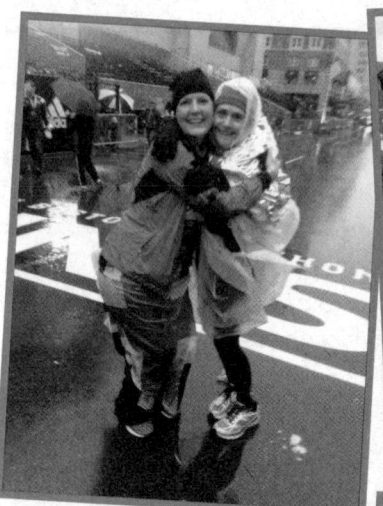
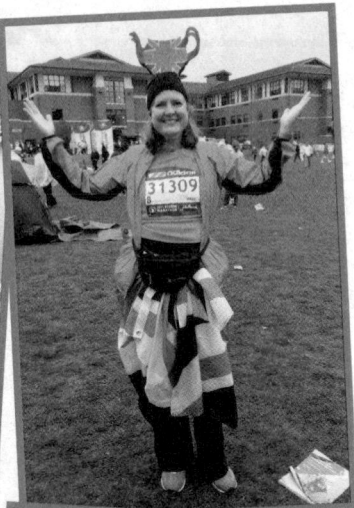
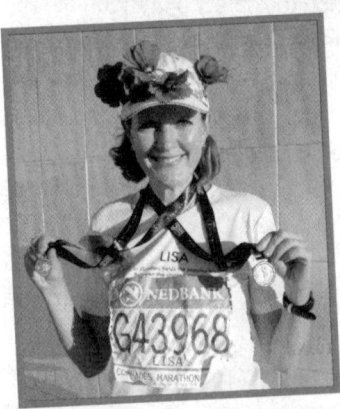
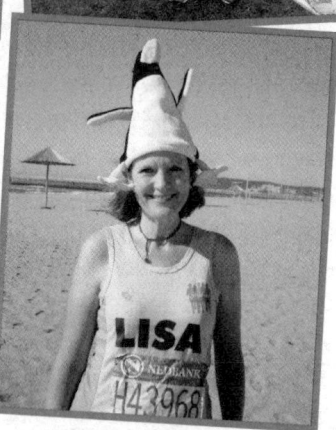
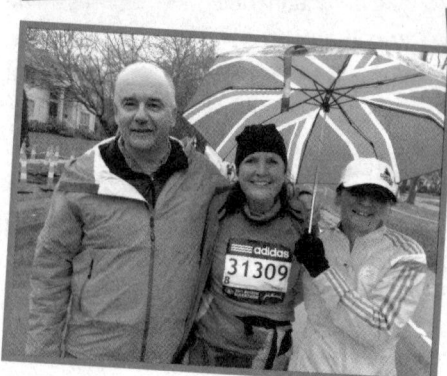
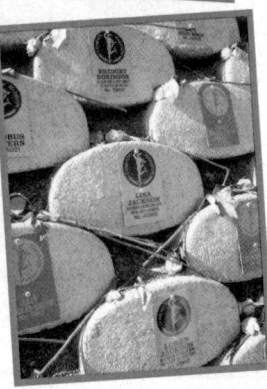

Chapter 8

What running taught me about... failure and success

> Failures, repeated failures, are finger posts on the road to achievement. One fails forward toward success
>
> C. S. Lewis

If there's one thing you should know about me it's that I don't 'do' failure. Ever since childhood I've always aimed to succeed at everything I put my mind to – and if I wasn't likely to succeed I sure as hell wasn't even going to try. Running changed that. When I became a runner I simply had to embrace the risk that sometimes I wouldn't be going home with a medal. I had no idea whether I'd be able to complete my first marathon, but I did – and my self-belief skyrocketed.

However, even though I now knew that I could definitely go the distance, each successive marathon was such a struggle that there *still* weren't any guarantees I'd finish. Now that I've done dozens of marathons, they're a lot less daunting. I've learned to listen to my body and distinguish between the times when it's saying 'Ahem, don't mean to bother you, but I think you may be experiencing something we experts call pain' (said in a quiet voice, which just means my muscles are working hard) and 'OH GOD THAT HURTS!' (screamed almost out loud, meaning that I should stop moving *immediately* or risk tearing or breaking something). I've learned to disregard the former – and, of course, heed the latter. However, these days I'm facing a new challenge: being able to finish within the cut-offs. This means that, 16 years after my first one, every marathon continues to be oh-so-subtly tinged with a fear of failure. But having felt the fear and run with it over and over again I've learned not to let it stop me from starting.

You'd think that the fact I'd come to terms with the possibility of failing would make failing, when it happened, easier to bear. It hasn't. Each time I fail to achieve a running goal it comes as a huge shock. Denial, anger, bargaining, depression – I still have to go through every single one of the stages of grief before I'm able to accept what's occurred and move on. But what I've learned from failing has surprised me and delighted me. Because, like coming last in a race, far from being the worst thing that can happen, it can often be the best.

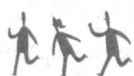

When I first ran the Comrades Marathon in 2009 I prayed I'd finish in time – if I hadn't made it on my first attempt I'd never have been prepared to put myself through all that taxing training again. So when I met Amit Sheth that year, a runner who'd failed to complete Comrades more times than he'd finished it, I was full of admiration. I encountered Amit again when I returned to South Africa the following year to claim my 'back-to-back' Comrades medal, a commemorative medal given to runners who do their first and second Comrades in consecutive years. In the intervening year he'd authored a book called *Dare to Run* chronicling the journey he and his wife Neepa had taken to become the first Indian husband and wife duo to complete Comrades. In 2010 I knew I simply had to succeed: this was my only chance to win two medals – the standard Comrades Marathon one, and the back-to-back one – in one go; a once-in-a-lifetime two-for-one offer.

The race traditionally reverses direction every year, but because 2010's event coincided with South Africa's hosting of the FIFA World Cup, for the first time in its history it was run in the same direction two years in a row as Durban provided a bigger venue than Pietermaritzburg for the 100,000 spectators who were expected to be at the finish to welcome the larger-than-usual number of participants home. Hence I'd be running the same downhill route I'd conquered the year before. My husband Graham had found spectating at Comrades for 12 hours so boring that he'd been persuaded to run it with me, so once again I had a training buddy. With my newfound confidence (read cockiness) from finishing Comrades the year before despite doing far less training than I'd been advised to do, I did about half of the recommended training this time round and replaced the suggested three ultras and two marathons in three months with a plan of my own: running three marathons in 15 days, which I duly did, with London being a lifetime PB of 4h38.

Come Comrades day, I coasted to the finish two minutes faster than I had the year before despite not being able to keep up with my friend Bridget, who'd done almost 100 per cent of the training and hence ran a fabulous debut Comrades in 10h42. 'I've cracked this Comrades thing!' I remember thinking jubilantly. The hamstring injury I'd sustained during the ultra I'd done while training for my previous Comrades proved to me that it was far more important to arrive at the start undertrained but uninjured rather than well-trained and injured. And that for those of us who simply wanted to finish, Comrades training really didn't need to be as scarily intimidating or intense as most programmes suggested.

Besides hugging Graham and Bridget at the finish and sharing their joy in being awarded their first Comrades medals, my favourite memory of that year's race is somewhat unorthodox. It isn't every day – in all honesty, it's only happened once – that someone has asked to photograph my bottom. Actually, it's a part of me I tend to avoid aiming at cameras as it's more Kim Kardashian than perky Pippa Middleton. So I was startled when, very early on in the race, a male runner tapped my shoulder and enquired whether he could take a picture of my bottom on his mobile phone, promising to send it to me if I gave him my email address. 'I'm not trying to make a pass at you,' he explained, looking rather embarrassed. 'It's just that I've never seen a running tuckshop before!' It was my idiosyncratic running belt that had attracted his attention. I've never been a gel gal so instead had come up with my own idea of what constituted appropriate race-day nutrition: thin little strips of dried beef called biltong (a South African delicacy that resembles an expensive dog treat), plenty of chocolate and an assortment of multicoloured protein bars, each stuffed into the little elasticated loops of my gel belt. I looked less like a well-prepared, seasoned marathon runner and more like a ridiculous caricature of Rambo who, armed only with an abundance of food, planned to eat her way through the coming mission.

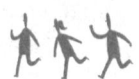

They say pride comes before a fall, and it really does. The following year I was back at Comrades for the third time to tackle the notorious Up run from Durban on the coast to Pietermaritzburg in the hinterland, a course where the first 37K (23 miles) involves running uphill almost continuously. In those days it wasn't necessary to requalify if you'd finished Comrades the previous year so I hadn't worried too much about trying to run marathons in under five hours. I also hadn't been too concerned about hill training – I mean, I'd already done Comrades *twice*; I was now a veteran. 'The more you sweat in training, the less you bleed in battle.' That piece of advice didn't apply to me, I thought. My training volume dropped still further to about 40 per cent of the 1,200K (745 miles) suggested.

I vividly recall standing at the start line at 5.30am with my friend Bridget and my husband Graham, both of whom were aiming for their back-to-back medals. Graham's last words to me before he headed off to his own (faster) start pen were: 'Good luck. And don't go tripping over any cat's eyes.' Then we were off, 16,000 people shuffling quietly through Durban's darkened streets. Unlike the Down run there was no cheerful chatter – the idea that we'd be tackling a course where the total elevation gain was 1,166 m (3,825 ft) (the equivalent of running up Cape Town's Table Mountain and then some) was really daunting. I was extremely apprehensive as I hadn't run for three weeks due to having very painful calves. In fact, I was unsure that I'd even be able to run a half marathon, let alone 87K (54 miles) that day.

Disaster struck just after the '86KM TO GO' sign (unlike most races, the distance markers in Comrades scarily proclaim the distance you have yet to cover, not how far you've already run). I tripped on a cat's eye and fell heavily onto my left elbow and left knee. Instantly, two runners hooked their arms through mine and hauled me back onto my feet: if they hadn't scooped me up so quickly I would've been trampled by the thousands of runners behind us. I was in utter shock from the intensity of the pain and I immediately thought of pulling out, but I had invested too much to quit after just one kilometre. Not only was there the financial investment (flying from London to South Africa and back) and the physical investment in my training (even if it was less than suggested), but I had also overcome a virus, two colds and the flu, healed an injured knee and had numerous sports-massage and physio sessions to get myself race-ready. To snap myself out of it, I kept saying out loud: 'I'm fine, I'm going to be fine,' until I started to believe it. All I remember thinking is that it felt as if my arm had almost been torn off. If you think of twisting a drumstick to detach it from a chicken carcass you'll get the picture of the trauma inflicted on my shoulder. Bleeding profusely, I tried to keep up with Bridget in the 12-hour pacing group but I soon realised I simply couldn't maintain their pace, and so Bridget and I parted company.

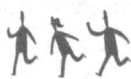

To stay motivated I kept setting myself small targets: first I aimed to do a half marathon, then to reach Hillcrest where I knew my supporters would be waiting (my sister's exhortation to 'Keep calm – and keep going!' buoyed my spirits no end), then to complete at least a marathon, then to reach the halfway mark before the 6h10 cut-off. I was secretly hoping I'd miss the cut-off and be forced to withdraw but I got there with about seven minutes to spare and so was duty bound to continue. Soon afterwards I was able to fulfil my main goal for this Comrades: to scatter my mother's ashes at the Wall of Honour. This beautiful landmark beside the route overlooks the Valley of a Thousand Hills and any runner who's successfully completed Comrades can purchase an oval-shaped concrete block and have a yellow or green plaque with their name on it attached to it. This year, among the wall's many new plaques, there was one bearing my name (and the words 'In loving memory of my Mom Leoné Jackson who will always be an inspiration'), one my sister's name and a third Bridget's.

On I went, chatting to many other runners who were suffering just as much, if not more, than me. One woman had vomited three times already that day; another was doing her first Comrades with her Dad and was mouthing 'Never again' all the way up Inchanga Hill. Every time a sweeper bus crawled by packed with ill and injured runners being ferried to the finish I looked at their faces, haggard from effort, haunted by failure, and asked myself the question: can I truly say I can't go a single step further? The answer was always: no. I resolved to continue moving forwards and walk with 'pride and purpose' as my (oft ignored but brilliant) training programme had instructed me.

Having covered 67K I came across Amit sprawled in the long grass at the side of the road waiting to board a sweeper bus to the finish. He'd had a bad case of food poisoning the day before and, even though I suggested he accompany me, was too weak to continue. By this stage I knew there was no hope of finishing before the 12-hour cut-off but I also knew there was no way

I would bail – I grinned as I told myself they'd have to catch me, tie my ankles together and throw me in the bus headfirst before I'd surrender. And so I kept pressing on past the fields of impossibly green sugar cane. For the final half hour I struggled my way up Polly Shortts, the last of Comrades' legendary Big Five hills, accompanied by a convoy of about 20 sweeper buses, ambulances, paramedic vehicles and police cars, the latter needlessly dramatically flashing their lights.

I persevered until 5.32pm when two officials suddenly sprung out of a car and told me, very categorically, that my race was over. Footsore and covered in streaks of dried blood, sweat and tears I gratefully sat down in the minibus, having covered 78.5K (48.8 miles). But my odyssey was not over: just a few hundred metres down the road an elderly runner steadfastly refused to get into the bus, knowing that only race officials had the power to force him to withdraw from the race. Since none were in sight, he gamely plodded on for the next 90 minutes or so, with all 20 vehicles trailing behind him like a slow-motion presidential cavalcade. Fortunately I was able to borrow a phone to let my family know I was safe or else they'd have been worried sick. When we eventually reached the medical tent at the finish I dragged myself out of the bus, took five steps and promptly passed out. When I came to, I could taste grass in my mouth and was staring at the ankles of half a dozen medics.

My appointed doctor threatened me with a drip, but after all I'd been through that was one challenge too far (I've always hated needles) and I adamantly refused. My 'punishment' was being forced to sip ten cups of sparkling orange drink – and having to prove I didn't have kidney damage by going to the loo. Eventually I managed both and got discharged at 9pm.

And so my third Comrades ended in 'failure'. I didn't get a medal or an official time. But I did get a great day full of unforgettable experiences, and that night we joyfully celebrated Graham and Bridget both being given back-to-back medals. I did have a moment of personal glory the next day, however, when, thanks to my jaunty-looking penguin hat, photos of me were published in two local newspapers.

Comrades was the first race I'd ever 'failed' to finish. It took me a long time to come to terms with it. I felt gutted at not finishing, but elated that I hadn't taken the easy way out and bailed after the first kilometre when I had the chance. I felt proud that I'd stuck it out to the bitter end like I said I would. I didn't know it then but my running career would give me several other opportunities to experience what many people would call 'failure'. In the coming years running was going to teach me that 'failure' and 'success' are not necessarily mutually exclusive. Receiving a medal is undoubtedly fabulous but it's definitely not the only measure of a 'successful' race.

After Comrades I asked Bridget what our next challenge should be, only to be taken aback by her answer: 'Boston!' The world's oldest annual marathon also has the world's most fearsomely fast qualifying times. This was the equivalent of asking Bridget what she'd like to do after retirement and her responding: 'Become a lion tamer.' But Bridget isn't someone whose dreams I wanted to stamp on and when she sent me an email detailing the times we'd need to achieve to qualify I dutifully pasted a printout onto the noticeboard in my study. In 2011, before the qualifying times were made even more eyeballs-out fast, a woman aged 40 to 44 needed to run a marathon in under 3h50. For me this meant slicing a whopping 48 minutes from my PB. I'd done it before (and more!) when I'd gone from 5h54 in Dublin to 4h39 in Seville, but could I do it again? Research revealed that some runners had made no fewer than 15 attempts to qualify for Boston, so I did what Mark Twain did whenever he got the urge to exercise: lie down until the feeling passed. In my case this involved resolving to wait to grow older, as women aged 45 and over were allowed an additional ten minutes.

My forty-fifth birthday came and went. Every now and again Bridget would mention the Boston dream and, as my times were heading in the opposite direction, I'd tell her I'd think about it. But deep down I thought it was impossible.

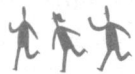

That was until the day a woman called Kathrine Switzer bounded into my life. I'd been eager to interview her ever since I'd seen the 1967 photos of her fending off an angry race official who'd tried to tear off her race number and boot her off the Boston Marathon course. It's not very often you see a woman in a baggy tracksuit being chased mid-race by a balding man in a blazer with a snarl on his face. I've always been proud to call myself a feminist so I found it utterly incomprehensible that women weren't allowed to enter marathons in 1967, the year I was born. Apparently, women were considered too weak physically – it was feared the wombs of us delicate ladies would drop out, or that running would make us too manly – which is why that race official attempted to evict the 20-year-old journalism student who'd entered the race using the gender-neutral name of KV Switzer. What the official hadn't counted on was Kathrine's beefy boyfriend Tom, an aspiring Olympic hammer thrower, who barged him out of the way. Kathrine defiantly completed the marathon and went on to campaign for all women to enter, not just the Boston Marathon, but *all* marathons. Eventually she even succeeded in ensuring the acceptance of the women's marathon into the 1984 Olympic Games.

In preparation for our interview, I took Kathrine's autobiography, *Marathon Woman*, on holiday to Mexico with me and, having flopped onto a sunlounger, began reading about her remarkable life. The book was packed with hilarious anecdotes (Kathrine ran her first Boston with a sanitary bag containing dextrose sweets wrapped round her wrist) and I drove my husband to distraction by insisting on reading out the 'best bits' to him every five minutes.

By the time I'd finished reading her book I felt I'd made a new friend so I couldn't wait to Skype Kathrine, and what was supposed to be a 20-minute interview turned into a two-hour chat. And that 'little chat' brought me to the start line of the Boston Marathon. Getting to know Kathrine, and twice running the fabulous 261 Women's Marathon in Majorca (which is named after her famous bib number and which she hosted personally), reignited my desire to run Boston, and prompted me to secure a press place to cover it for *Women's Running* magazine.

Getting a media place meant I didn't need to run a qualifying time to gain entry to the 2015 Boston Marathon. It also meant that I felt like an imposter when I arrived to collect my race number. While walking through Boston Common I kept spotting little herds of runners trotting hither and thither: it was as if I'd stumbled into an army base where everyone runs in formation, even to fetch a pint of milk. Boston has ferociously fast qualifying times – even 80-year-old women are expected to be able to finish a marathon in 5h25, whereas women like myself aged 45 to 49 have to run in under 3h55 – so simply everyone looked mean, keen and extremely lean. Suffering from feet so outrageously painful they'd flummoxed my physio, I wasn't entirely sure of my chances of finishing within the six-hour cut-off, but I wasn't going to let a small thing like that stop me from following in Kathrine's footsteps. The rules of the 100 Marathon Club state that you can add any marathon or ultramarathon to your tally, provided it's an official race and as long as your name appears in the results list, no matter if your time was outside the cut-off. I'd hurriedly researched the results from the previous year and had seen that runners with times well over six hours had been given official finishing times, so I was cautiously optimistic that this marathon would count towards my 100 Marathon Club membership. But what I wasn't sure of was whether these runners had been given a time because they were all in their 70s and 80s. Would they also bend the rules for an injured 40-something? I'd have to suck it and see.

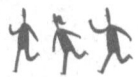

Boston is arguably the most famous marathon on the planet so I found it charming that the race actually has a kind of school-sports-day feel. And it's not just the big fleet of little yellow school buses that ferry runners to the start line in Hopkinton that gives it this atmosphere: it's the town of Hopkinton itself, all little clapboard houses with wide lawns and Snoopy mailboxes set among trees. We'd been warned to expect the kind of wet and windy weather Kathrine had encountered 48 years before, and for once the weathermen had got it right. The minute we stepped off the bus the downpour started, and it didn't let up all day. Huddled under the big-top-like marquee on the sports field of the local high school, alongside many runners dressed in the old clothes, pyjamas and dressing gowns they'd worn to ward off the cold but would discard at the start line, I felt more like a refugee than a runner. There wasn't any of the cheery banter I'm used to at marathon starts: these were extremely serious runners for whom running was an extremely serious business. Hence, when I draped myself in a huge Union Jack and donned the cardboard teapot headgear that would turn me into the Boston Tea Party, for the first time in my running life I felt strangely ridiculous. Unlike all the other Marathon Majors I'd run, fancy dress just wasn't what people did at Boston. Remember the scene in *Bridget Jones's Diary* where she turns up at a posh party dressed as a Playboy bunny? That was me.

I was in the fourth wave, so at about 11am I made my way in the direction of the start line. Running downhill for the first few miles felt glorious. What made this gentle descent even more special was the fact that the route was along a narrow road and that, even though it was pelting it down, the citizens of Hopkinton had come out to shout encouragement and shake cowbells at us while sheltering under their beach umbrellas and garden gazebos. I was really surprised that, unlike city marathons that are invariably held on huge highways or broad boulevards, Boston, for all its prestige, felt a little homespun, like a tea cosy your gran may have knitted.

Just 1K into the race I had to head to the loo, and when I emerged there were hardly any other runners left on the course and I steeled myself for a silent slog. It didn't help that my cardboard teapot had now become sodden and had collapsed, forcing me to throw it away. I was no longer the Boston Tea Party but a woman in a giant, soaking-wet Union Jack. I hoped Bostonians had short memories because most of their history involved fighting the British, not cheering for them. I needn't have worried: the little signs they'd staked into their front lawns saying 'Smile if you're not wearing underwear' and 'Run, stranger, run' said it all.

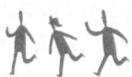

For a few more miles the route continued through the forested New England countryside, passing some of the 100,000 daffodils planted as signs of hope and defiance after the bombings of 2013 and giant posters proclaiming: 'Only in Boston do a million people take the day off so 30,000 can work.' The latter was a reference to the fact that the race is held on the third Monday in April, Patriots' Day, which is a public holiday in the state of Massachusetts.

On the shore of Lake Cochituate I ran for a mile or so with Dave Clark, an American runner who was running his fourth Boston... that day! He'd already run to and from Boston three times and was on his final 26.2.

'What drugs are you on?' I enquired incredulously.

'It's more about the drugs I'm *not* on,' said Dave, who told me he'd written a book about his journey from obese alcoholic (who often downed two bottles of Scotch a day) to vegan ultrarunner.

A little further on, in the town of Natick, I met kindergarten teacher and mum-of-four Kim Shamah, who'd been prevented from finishing Boston in 2013 when the bombs went off and had withdrawn from the 2014 event because she'd been diagnosed with ovarian cancer.

'I told my oncologist, "I don't care what you have to do but you're getting me to the start line of the 2015 Boston Marathon,"' she said.

I noticed that Kim had little circular badges pinned to her beanie and asked her if she was running in honour of someone.

'Yes, a close friend who died of cancer – she drew the pictures on my badges as she was a talented artist.' As we pushed on through the rain, Kim shared that she was not just doing Boston for that friend but also to celebrate another friend who was in remission from breast cancer, and in memory of her dad who'd died of cancer. I shared how my mum and aunt had also died before their time, and at the same moment we both burst into tears. Now it *really* got hard to keep going – our choking sobs were badly affecting our breathing. I felt nothing but sadness, aware only of the huge hole our lost loved ones had left in our lives. Tears mixed with sweat mixed with rain.

Just then we arrived at Wellesley College, one of the most prestigious women's liberal-arts colleges in the US. But their academic prowess isn't what these ladies are best known for. They have two other major claims to fame: cheering and kissing. Even though it was three-and-a-half hours since the front runners had passed by they were still out in force, eager to maintain their reputation for puckering up, whatever the weather.

'Kiss me, I'm from Oregon!' read a poster one of them held up. 'Kiss me, I'm from China!' said another.

'Kiss me, I have an umbrella!'

'Kiss me, I have a great personality!'

And my favourite: 'Kiss me, I left the library for you!'

We were kept so busy laughing that our crying miraculously stopped, but Kim soon started again when her family, including her husband Steve, unexpectedly emerged from the sidelines and began hugging her. Eight hugs later we were on our way again, cheered on by a marshal wearing headgear that resembled an umbrella mixed with a frilly floral bathing hat.

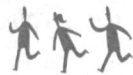

On we trudged, passing another group holding up a sign saying 'It's Boston, Bitches – Run Faster!' If only we could! We kept passing and getting passed by Richard Carling, a Utah State Senator dressed in a neon-orange cap and shorts. No sooner would we pass him than we'd need a loo break and so he'd sneak past us again.

'How many times have you gone to the loo today?' I asked Kim while exiting a Portaloo and trying for the umpteenth time to awkwardly yank up my two pairs of sodden and hence sticky running tights.

'I've actually lost count,' she said.

We got chatting to the senator and learned that he was running Boston for the thirty-seventh time – and that he was

77 years old. 'You're doing great,' he kept reassuring us as we battled the headwinds that were now punching us in the face with endless uppercuts.

And then I saw what would prove to be the most emotional sight of a day full of emotional moments. A group of people were walking shoulder to shoulder up ahead of us. As we drew closer we could see that they were the support crew for a frail-looking runner who'd take a few faltering steps, rest for a few seconds, and then take a few more.

Kim and I shouted our good wishes as we passed, little knowing that whereas our race would end at around 6pm that evening his would end at 5am the next morning, and that he'd not only have to survive 20 hours on his feet but the massive thunderstorm that would lash Boston that night. We didn't know it then, but despite having muscular dystrophy, Maickel Melamed would be the race's final finisher.

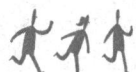

After a few more miles it was my turn to shed a tear for the second time as my own two personal cheerleaders – Helly and Ted – appeared in the distance, holding the Union Jack umbrella they'd promised to bring so I could spot them more easily. I'd met Helly – a Brit living in Boston – at the halfway mark of the Chicago Marathon six months before and she'd saved me from what had been a surprisingly lonely race. Helly hadn't actually intended to do more than the first 2K of Chicago, and was only doing that to keep her marathon-virgin husband Ted company: an injured thigh had meant she hadn't run for six weeks, she was suffering from a nasty head cold and hadn't eaten any carbs the night before. But thanks to the power of chat we'd made it all the way to Grant Park, held hands as we finished and shared the most heavenly pint of ice-cold beer moments later. Helly had certainly lived up to the motto printed on her T-shirt: 'I run for beer, wine and tea.' When I learned that I was coming to Boston I'd immediately contacted her and she'd promised to be there to support me. What I didn't suspect then was that supporting me would involve standing in the rain for *five hours*.

'You really didn't have to,' I said. 'This weather is so foul I definitely didn't expect you to come.'

'Nonsense,' she replied. 'We said we'd be here, so here we are. Get under the umbrella.'

'It's too late,' I said. 'There's a stream of water running down the *inside* of my knickers! It's better if you use it to keep yourselves dry.'

Gabbling away happily as we pressed on, I introduced Kim and Senator Carling to my friends, and then, after about 20 minutes, I abruptly stopped.

'Hold on a minute, Helly,' I said. 'Where's Heartbreak Hill? You said you'd meet me on Heartbreak Hill.'

'Oh sweetheart,' she laughed. 'We *did* meet you on Heartbreak, that's about a mile back along the road.'

'What?' I shrieked. 'You mean I missed it? That was it? The most notorious hill in the whole marathon-running world and I missed it?'

''Fraid so,' said Helly. 'It's actually not that steep but it can be a killer as it comes just after you've run twenty miles downhill and aren't really expecting it.'

I wasn't sure whether to be relieved that the worst was over or cheesed off that I hadn't had the opportunity to photograph it.

And then I started chuckling, because I realised I'd once again inadvertently followed in Kathrine's footsteps more literally than I'd intended to. She too had run Boston on a day so raw the wind felt like a razor, a day so wet that there were puddles inside her shoes. She too had worn lipstick. And she too had got to the top of Heartbreak without noticing it, having, like me, expected, as she wrote in her book, 'that there would be a trumpet herald or something at the top'. Her coach Arnie had told her she had to be the only person not to have known they'd just run over Heartbreak Hill. Well, I was the second! The fearsome Heartbreak Hill may have been conquered, but I was getting increasingly anxious as time went by that we were going to be pulled off the course as there were so few runners on the road ahead of us. Each time we saw a policeman I avoided making eye contact in case he had been instructed to bundle us into a sweeper van and drive us to the finish.

'Whatever we do we need to keep that senator in our sights,' I told Kim. 'There's no way they're going to stop him from finishing his thirty-seventh Boston, so as long as we can pretend that he needs our support I think they'll let us finish, too.' This proved much harder than expected as Senator Carling was not only a strong runner, but didn't make as many loo stops as we did. I lost Kim at one of them: when I emerged she was nowhere in sight but I could see the senator's orange cap in the distance so I sprinted to catch up with him. I was incredibly glad that I managed to, eventually, as his tales of starting marathon running at 40 were so inspiring – and to think I'd always considered myself a late starter at 31.

At long last we spotted the red triangle of the famous CITGO sign near the legendary Fenway Park baseball ground. Just one mile to go. The senator and I picked up speed. Then a sharp right turn into Hereford Street.

'This is where the police turned me back during the bombings,' he said.

Another sharp turn left into Boylston Street and we were on the home straight.

'Right, time to finish this thing,' I said to the senator, grabbing his hand. Then all of a sudden Kim's husband was hugging me.

'Great to see you again, Steve,' I cried, 'but just let me finish first.'

'You've *already* finished!' said Steve.

'What?' I looked around in confusion: in the driving rain I couldn't quite work out where we were. Where were the international flags I'd recalled seeing in photos of the finish? In most marathons you run under a finish arch with a huge clock on it, whereas here the photo bridge was still up ahead.

'We can't have,' I said. 'Where's the finish line?'

'There,' he said, pointing to the huge yellow letters painted onto the road a few metres behind us which I'd already run over but had failed to notice. I raised my arms jubilantly in the air and let out a whoop. I couldn't quite believe it. After running in what felt like a car wash for seven hours we'd got there. I had finished the world's most prestigious marathon.

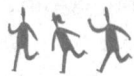

Shivering uncontrollably, I was so cold by the time I got back to my hostel that I couldn't attend the marathon after-party in Fenway Park. Nor could I go out on the town, where I later heard many runners were bought free drinks by admiring

Bostonians. I was chilled to the bone and it took me 30 minutes in a hot shower to thaw out. But I'd done it, I'd run Boston! Despite the fact that the conditions had been appalling, it had most definitely exceeded all my expectations.

Curled up in bed with my medal round my neck I stumbled across a section in my guidebook that described Henry David Thoreau's 26-month stay in a simple cabin in the woods near Boston in an attempt to 'live deliberately'. He'd written a book about this experience called *Walden*, in which he explained that he'd conducted this experiment in order to 'live deep and suck out all the marrow of life'. My 26 miles through Massachusetts – one for every month Thoreau spent at Walden Pond – had given me, too, the chance to live deliberately. For one glorious day I'd experienced almost every emotion imaginable: sadness over those killed and maimed by the Boston bombings and for my mother and aunt whose deaths meant they'd never run beside me again; admiration for those running despite the odds stacked against them; fear at not being allowed to finish; gratitude for those willing to brave a blowing gale to urge us onwards; and elation at finally reaching that famous yellow FINISH and being presented with a medal.

The next day I got an email from my husband saying he couldn't find my finishing time online. An anguished hour on the computer followed as I tried to locate it. It wasn't there. The year before the organisers had recorded the time of everyone who finished, even if they hadn't made the official six-hour cut-off, and published it on the Boston Marathon website, but this year they hadn't. I felt a real sense of grief. Boston had been one of the most gruelling marathons I'd ever run and not to have a time or have it count towards my 100 Marathon Club membership was devastating. But, as always, my husband saved the day. 'Lisa,' he emailed me, 'you didn't go to Boston to get a time, you went there to have an experience. And judging by what you've told me, you've most certainly done that!'

I spent the rest of my time in Boston trying to remember the truth of Graham's words and shake off the horrible feeling of having failed, which lingered even after I returned home. I even pulled out of a marathon I was due to do the week I got back as I simply couldn't cope with two DNFs (Did Not Finish) in one week. And then, several months later, when my Comrades friend Barbara was reading the first draft of this book, for some unknown reason she took it upon herself to once again look for my time online. Miraculously it was now there, and she immediately emailed me the good news. Granted it was an estimated time, but it was still a time. Shaking with excitement I contacted Traviss, the Chairman of the 100 Marathon Club – would he accept an estimated time? Turned out he would. And so what had felt like my biggest failure turned into one of my biggest triumphs. I could, after all, proudly count Boston towards my 100-marathon goal.

So what has running taught me about failure and success? Rudyard Kipling once wrote, 'If you can meet with Triumph and Disaster/And treat those two impostors just the same… Yours is the Earth and everything that's in it/And – which is more – you'll be a Man, my son!' I take this to mean that success and failure are often interchangeable. On many occasions running has taught me that Rudyard was right. For instance, the very first time I came last in a marathon was at the super-tough South Downs Marathon – but I got to hug a friend in a chest-high bean field and spend a whole day in some of the most 'ahh'-some scenery England has to offer. Failure? I don't think so. I failed to finish the Bacchus Marathon one year because my calf muscle tore – but I succeeded in finishing it two years later. I may have been asked to withdraw halfway through the Portsmouth Coastal Waterside Marathon for being too slow, but I negotiated an earlier start time the following year with the friendly race director and so, spurred on by my initial 'failure', I completed my unfinished business with that race, too. On the other hand, I succeeded in achieving a PB of 4h38 in the 2010 London Marathon but I failed to speak to a single other runner during the race, making it less enjoyable than many other marathons I've run, demonstrating that 'success' and 'failure' are in fact very subjective.

All of this has made me realise that, while the running columnist John 'The Penguin' Bingham was correct when he wrote that the miracle wasn't that he finished, but that he had the courage to start, what running has really given me is the courage to *fail*. To begin the journey but accept that it won't always necessarily end in success. And so I'll continue to run even when some people will dismissively call what I do 'jogging'. I'll continue to have a good giggle when someone, on hearing how often I come last, remarks that I should write to running apparel manufacturers suggesting they pay me *not* to run in their gear. In fact, I'll continue coming last, as I've done in 19 other marathons since that day on the South Downs, because it's way better than not turning up at all. My headstone isn't going to say: 'Here lies Lisa Jackson. She watched every hot new box set. Twice.' It'll read: 'Here lies Lisa Jackson. Marathoner. Trailrunner. Triathlete. Ultrarunner. She's reached the final finishing line – and this time, she isn't last.'

'There is no failure, only feedback'

'I attempted the Comrades ultramarathon three times – and finished only once'

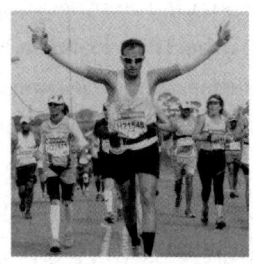

'Dear God, why me, why now?' These must have been Paula Radcliffe's thoughts as she sat sobbing on an Athenian kerbside having pulled out of the 2004 Olympic women's marathon at the 21-mile mark. And at the 67K mark of the 2011 Comrades ultramarathon they were my thoughts too, as I lay on the roadside waiting for the bus that ferries injured and exhausted runners to the finish. The day before a stomach bug had flushed all the nutrients from my body and no amount of mental strength could have got me through the remaining 22 kilometres in the two hours and 20 minutes left before the 12-hour cut-off. I simply didn't have the energy to get going again, even when Lisa came past and offered to accompany me, saying we shouldn't stop until we were forced to do so by the officials. I knew God didn't have time to worry about Comrades runners not finishing, especially when the world is full of far greater misery: death, disease and poverty. And I was also aware that I never ask God, 'Why me, why now?' when things go right – it's only the bad stuff He has to account for. But I did wonder if there was a karmic reason, as opposed to a purely scientific one, for my not finishing. Did I do something to *deserve* a DNF?

I didn't run for a month after Comrades as the DNF still troubled me. I'd lined up on the start line three times and reached the finish only once. One out of three is pretty bad. And then I realised I was asking the wrong questions. I shouldn't have been asking 'Why me, why now?' but '*What* now?' I decided I'd moped enough and that it was time to start getting ready for Comrades 2012. It was time to strap on my Garmin and head out the door. And you know what? I did.

Amit Sheth, 48, Mumbai, India

In 2012, Amit successfully completed the Comrades Marathon for the second time in 11h57.

'I failed at running a barefoot marathon in Antarctica'

Running barefoot started out as a dare on 30 December 2012 when I was preparing to run my fifth marathon in five days, my fiftieth that year. I'd brought only four pairs of minimalist Vibram FiveFingers running shoes and each pair is good only for a single marathon before needing to be washed because of the stench.

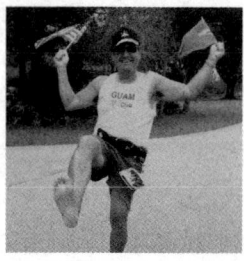

I joked with the other runners that I didn't have any shoes to wear for my final marathon and that I might have to run totally barefoot. They dared me to go ahead, so I did, dedicating my first barefoot marathon to my late parents. It was my way of allowing them to be part of my journey and I wanted them there to give me strength every step of the way. I have been running barefoot on and off ever since.

One of the first things I noticed while running barefoot was that simply everyone wanted to know whether my feet hurt, and I'd usually respond jokingly: 'Only when I think about it.' That usually made them smile – but also made them feel guilty when they realised they'd just made me think about it. I do still feel the pain of stepping on sharp rocks and running in freezing temperatures but I've become used to it (and it helps that my calluses have gotten thicker).

I enjoyed my first barefoot marathon and the attention that it created so much that I decided to use it for a good cause. I chose Soles4Souls, a charity that provides shoes to some of the 300 million kids worldwide who're too poor to afford adequate footwear. To compound the problem, most countries, like the Philippines, where I was born, don't allow children to attend school unless they wear shoes and this contributes to the vicious cycle of poverty. Since that first barefoot marathon I've completed a total of 208 full marathons and ultras in 13 different countries, 124 of them barefoot. Along the way I've raised over $13,000 to fund 13,000 pairs of shoes.

To maximise the amount of money raised I succeeded in breaking two Guinness World Records in 2014: 'Most barefoot marathons run on consecutive days (male)' (I ran ten) and 'Most barefoot marathons run in one year' (I ran 101). I'm also the first and only person to have completed 50 marathons in 50 US states barefoot, and have done a marathon on all seven continents, six of them barefoot.

My secret weapon is my trusty pair of tweezers. I've put them to good use on several occasions, such as when I ran the Day of the Dead Marathon in New Mexico. It was a 12-lap course littered with the incredibly prickly burrs of puncturevine plants and I stepped on about 50 of them. I had to keep sitting down and pulling them out with my tweezers.

It hasn't all gone without a hitch, however. There have been 19 marathons I didn't start and four I didn't finish. The former were mainly due to logistical issues such as flight delays and double bookings. A few injuries also resulted in my failing to finish some marathons, but my worst one occurred when I was hit by a car in Michigan. I could've been killed but I thankfully got away with just a few scratches.

In 2013 I attempted to become the first person to run a marathon barefoot in Antarctica but fell short of my goal. I was treading on some jagged rocks when the blisters on my right sole splattered blood all over my left foot. Less than a half mile later the blisters on my left foot burst as well. It was a long and excruciating trek back to base camp to get my feet cleaned and bandaged before I could finish the remaining 17.5 miles in shoes.

Despite having 'failed' in a few of my attempts, I've still run 2,646 miles (4,258 kilometres) barefoot and I'm not stopping anytime soon. As long as there are kids out there who need shoes, I'll keep running shoeless.

Eddie 'Barefoot Bandito' Vega, 55, North Carolina, USA

'Even barefooted Gandhi would've laughed at the state of my feet'

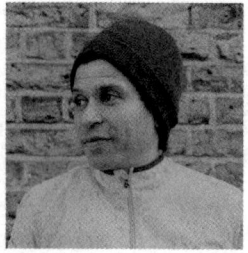

I always knew my feet were special but it wasn't until our first race that I fell head over heels in love with them. We were the dream team, my feet and I: fast, graceful and the envy of our running club. Those first few years were great as we shared sweaty frolics and heart-racing moments, spending hours running through muddy fields barely catching breath.

But it wasn't to last. Things changed. My feet changed. I don't know where we lost our love but waking up every morning to the sight of those gnarly goat hooves didn't help. Even the barefooted, mild-mannered Gandhi would've laughed at the state of my feet. The romance had died, date nights stopped, Vaseline Fridays were all but a distant memory. Even worse, my feet started to lose pace and we slipped further back down the pack.

To be honest, splitting up was never an option: I needed my feet to stand on and besides, I'd only just bought a new three-pack of value socks. So I tried everything to rekindle the love, including expensive shoes and a visit to a podiatrist, but that just left me out of pocket and still no closer to love.

Me and my feet are still together – but just as friends. Occasionally we put on our running shoes and waddle through the park for old times' sake. We don't break records, but it's nice. Who knows what the future holds and whether I'll ever get a second chance at love, but I'm here, waiting.

Taylor Huggins, 42, Croydon, London, England

In 2013 Taylor ran the Berlin Marathon in a time of 2h57 – and then, when his podiatrist diagnosed arthritis in his feet, he was forced to ditch running and became a bodybuilder. He soon realised this involved eating too much chicken and says he's now considering a career as an international gymnast. He still occasionally runs with Lisa's running club, Striders of Croydon.

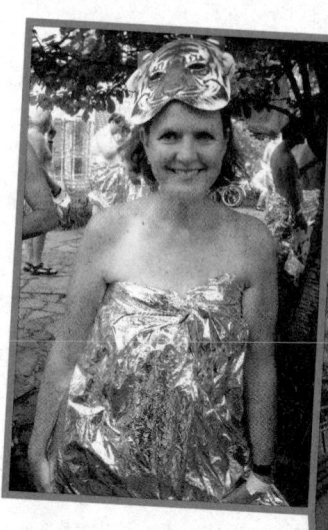

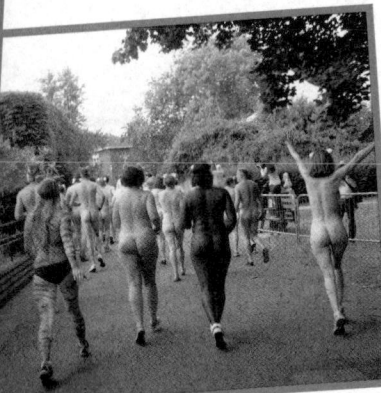

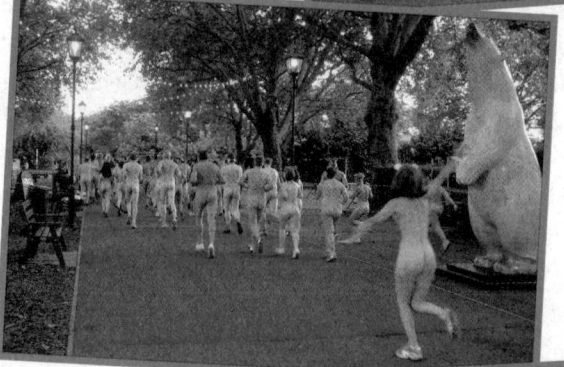

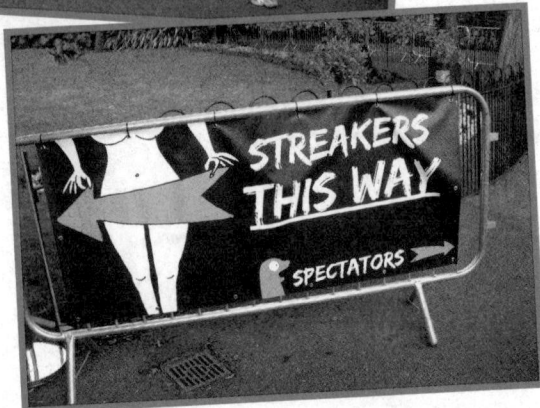

Chapter 9

What running taught me about... nudity

> I'm gonna put a curse on you and all your kids will be born completely naked
>
> Jimi Hendrix

I'd never experienced pre-race nerves quite like it: for a week I suffered sleepless nights, waking in the early hours in a cold sweat and then tossing and turning until morning. And even in daylight, whenever I thought of taking part I'd feel as if I'd been booted in the belly.

Only too soon race day dawned, and I lay in bed debating whether I should go or not. My husband was nowhere to be seen. He'd been so desperate to avoid participating that he'd signed up for a triathlon, the first event he'd ever entered himself (I usually book all our races and then tell him when it's too late for him to back out). Unfortunately, the race started at the respectable time of 11.30am so I couldn't use my standard 'Yikes, I overslept' excuse. Nor could I employ the 'It's too darn cold to run' one, as it was a gloriously warm spring day. And then came the clincher: this was one of only two such events within the whole of the UK (the other was hundreds of miles away in Wales), so if I was going to do it, it was now or never.

So what possessed me to run this totally terrifying 5K? It all started when I read Bart Yasso's book *My Life on the Run*, in which he described participating in a similar event. Bart is a legend in the US, where he's known as the Mayor of Running. US *Runner's World*'s Chief Running Officer, he's done over 1,000 races, including 200 marathons. I'd run most of the inaugural Jerusalem Marathon with Bart because the debilitating Lyme disease he has contracted has slowed him down considerably. Though not as much as you'd think: he left me at the 32K mark and still managed to beat my 5h38 finishing time by 28 minutes. Intrigued by his courage – and amazed by his tales of running the Badwater Marathon in Death Valley in temperatures that turned the tarmac into mush – I'd bought his book. And I found I had yet another reason to admire the man who'd run in both Antarctica and the Arctic, who'd outpaced a rhino in India and who'd twice cycled across America, alone, in just two weeks: he'd gone naked running. Now, usually when runners talk about 'naked running' they mean running without a watch or GPS – not Bart. He meant running without a watch, yes, but sans T-shirt, shorts and underwear, too, at a nudist camp in Washington State.

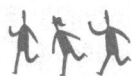

Inspired by Bart's cheeky run, I'd entered the BH5K Naked Run at The Naturist Foundation resort in Orpington, a leafy suburb in Kent. The reaction when I told my friends that I intended to run this race wasn't quite what I expected. No one asked me *why* I was going to do it, what they all wanted to know was *how*.

'What are you going to do about your boobs?' asked Michelle. 'Won't they jiggle about and be horribly uncomfortable?'

'I've no idea,' I replied. 'You'll probably be relieved to know I haven't run naked anywhere before.'

'Where are you going to pin your race number?' asked Teresa. 'Bet you haven't thought of that.'

No I hadn't, but I surmised I could run with it in one hand.

'You're going to run in Orpington? I was *born* in Orpington!' said another friend, Sue, no doubt imagining the horrified reaction of her former neighbours as they watched dozens of nudists bobbing past the half-timbered houses she remembered from her childhood.

'We'll be running *inside* a nudist resort – not on the high street,' I replied, chuckling.

'Are you going to run *completely* naked?' asked Christina, the then Editor of *Women's Running*.

'No, of course not,' I said, horrified. 'I'll be wearing socks and trainers.'

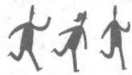

So that's how I ended up panicking in my bedroom on race morning, after a night of no sleep. The big debate raged in my head until, at 10.30am, I leapt up thinking, 'Screw it, let's do it,' and frantically crammed my kit into a holdall. This wasn't quite as simple a task as it sounds – what *does* one wear to a nudist camp? Thankfully, the organisers had sent me an email detailing naturist etiquette. It had informed me that 'one should always use a towel when seated (and naked)'. I couldn't quite work out the last bit. Surely, if you're wearing a towel, then you're not really naked? Having hastily dressed, and having left my bed unmade and a string of cupboards and drawers open, I grabbed a towel and a massive pot of Vaseline, snatched up my passport (to deter peeping Toms you have to provide photo ID) and hurtled out the door.

After typing the resort's postcode into my car's satnav I headed off. Of course I got hopelessly lost. Driving down the country lanes of deepest Kent I had no clue where I was. At long last I located the imposing gates of The Naturist Foundation and drew up alongside the intercom. But what was that I could see flitting through the trees at the top of the driveway? Yes, it was naked people. Naked people running through the woods. With dismay – and then a huge sense of relief – I realised that I'd missed the start of the race. But I'd already pushed the buzzer and was now on CCTV. My voice quavering with nerves I enquired whether the race had already started, knowing full well it had.

'Yes it has, but come on up to the clubhouse and we'll see what we can do,' said a very friendly female voice. Once there, I was greeted by the fully clothed receptionist who informed me that, although I'd missed the race start, I was welcome to stay and 'enjoy the facilities'.

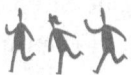

Just then another latecomer, Kim, arrived and we hit upon the idea of running the route on our own, once we'd watched the other participants finish. We went outside, still clothed, to cheer several dozen naked men across the finish line.

'A naked woman in heels is a beautiful thing,' the legendary French footwear designer Christian Louboutin once said, before adding, 'A naked man in shoes looks like a fool.' I have to agree with Christian: the male runners did look rather odd. But only at first. After spending five minutes applauding runners of all sizes, shapes and speeds as they sprinted past, we realised that the old adage still rings true: once you've seen one, you've seen 'em all.

We'd hoped to welcome the first lady home but the ladies were taking their time, so in the end we retired to the changing room where, naturally, there were no cubicles, just one huge horribly unisex empty room with a few lockers where men were getting changed. So we beat a retreat to the loos and, in what must have seemed like a game of speed strip poker, tore off our clothes and ran giggling outside, where the race director's wife lipsticked our race numbers onto our arms in a very fetching shade of fuchsia. After a quick explanation of the route we set off on a course that involved doing two-and-a-half laps around the grounds.

I have to say it was very comforting having Kim, a fellow nudie newbie, by my side as we passed little clusters of naked campers who cheered us as we trotted by.

'Well, it *is* a bit weird, don't you think?' Kim panted, as she led the way through the bluebell-bedecked woods.

'Mmm,' I pondered, as I chased her through the trees. 'It is… and it isn't. Running like this does put you in touch with nature, and it makes you wonder why we make such a fuss about wearing clothes.' My answer shocked me because only that morning I'd been convinced that I'd find every second of the experience lip-bitingly, toe-curlingly, bottom-clenchingly cringeworthy. It simply wasn't.

Thankfully, Michelle was wrong about my boobs – I'm quite flat-chested so failing to ban the bounce just wasn't an issue. But I have to admit I probably wouldn't want to run a marathon without wearing a sports bra. In fact, the only thing I wasn't OK with was my failure to apply Vaseline to my inner thighs. It wasn't long before my gait turned into a wide-legged waddle as the chafing began to take its toll. It gradually dawned on me that I'd most likely be spending the rest of the coming week walking as if I was smuggling a cheese-grater between my thighs.

We chat-ran our way round the course before retiring to the clubhouse for a hearty pub lunch and a cold beer. Yes, it was a bit weird queuing for a roast dinner with just a towel round my waist but what I found most unusual wasn't the fact that most people were naked but that they were so friendly. I'd never had so many strangers, both male and female, come up and talk to me in my life.

After lunch we lay on the lawn and topped up our tans alongside a 50-something maths professor who said he found naturism 'incredibly liberating' before relating how he'd participated in the World Naked Bike Ride through the streets of central London.

'Now *that* was tremendous fun,' he said, 'but I did have to ask the organisers to remove my photo from their website in case any of my students saw it.'

The race director's wife came over to chat, and informed us that of the 38 participants in the race only three had been women, and that one of them had walked all the way. Gutted, I realised that my late arrival had meant I'd missed out on probably my one and only chance to get a top place in a race.

As we were leaving Kim and I said farewell to the partner of a man we'd met in the lunch queue. What was most peculiar about her was that she was on her way to play tennis and had donned a sports bra. Kim and I agreed that the sight of this *half*-dressed woman, and not the waggling willies and bouncing boobs, was definitely the strangest sight we'd seen all day.

When I got home Graham was waiting for me, proudly wearing his triathlon medal.

'How was it?' he asked.

'Fine,' I said smiling.

'Did you almost chicken out?' he said with a grin.

'How did you know?'

'I took one look at all the open drawers and unmade bed and knew you'd left in a hurry.'

'OK, I'm busted,' I laughed. 'But I actually had a lot of fun and made a new friend. And it wasn't nearly as awkward as I'd imagined.' I told him that we had been invited back by the race director's wife for a jazz and real ale festival. 'Why don't you come with me? Just for the experience. Go on, please!'

Graham gave me a withering look, and then turned on his heels with a 'No'.

'Why not?' I said, pursuing him through the living room. 'There are going to be live bands and real ale – you *love* real ale.'

'No,' he said again.

'Honestly, it's a lovely place with a pool and woodlands and an outdoor gym.'

'I'm *not* going.'

'Why ever not?' I persisted.

'Because,' Graham said slowly, turning to face me, 'I don't like… jazz.'

There was no arguing with that.

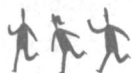

Fast-forward 13 weeks and I'm running naked round the grounds of London Zoo. This time I can't blame Bart but a relative who, upon hearing of my Orpington outing, sent me information about the forthcoming Streak for Tigers race. The event was held in support of the zoo's Sumatran Tiger campaign, and was based on the fact that a group of tigers is called a streak. The website promised a 350-metre circuit inside the zoo grounds with a mask and tiger ears thrown in for the camera shy. This was no ordinary discreet dash: the national press had been invited to witness the event.

Now, my first brush with naked running had taught me two things: one, you omit Vaseline at your peril and two, you don't want anyone you know seeing you do it, so I resolved to keep my clothes off – but my mask on.

The website's Q&A section handily covered the other thing I was worried about: law enforcement.

Question: Will I be arrested for nudity?

Answer: No. ZSL London Zoo is private land. However you must arrive and leave the event fully clothed.

Thank heavens for naturist etiquette.

And so I arrived at the suitably named Prince Albert Gate at London Zoo. There were about 300 of us tigers and some had really gone crazy and daubed themselves from head to toe in stripey bodypaint. After slipping into something more comfortable (my foil blanket, ears and mask) I headed outside where it was easy to spot the dyed-in-the-wool naturists as they'd 'forgotten' their blankets. The rest of us milled around making small talk while feeling rather apprehensive about discarding ours in a few minutes' time.

I got talking to Catherine, a tall 20-something-year-old. 'I'm not nearly as embarrassed as I thought I'd be,' she confided. 'But I suppose it's because we've all got boobs and we've all got… bits!'

Just before the start I was tapped on the shoulder by a male tiger in a foil blanket. 'Would you mind taking our photo?' he said, pointing to a similarly attired tigress whom he'd obviously only recently befriended. He handed over his smartphone which I wasn't sure how to operate.

'Does this thing need a flash?' I asked. They looked at each other, shrugged, and then said 'Yeah, sure,' and dropped their foil blankets to the ground. I belatedly realised they thought I'd said, 'Do you *want* to flash?'

Jettisoning our blankets, we raced out to greet the waiting cameras. It felt like the most natural thing in the world to be trotting round a zoo on a summer's evening as unencumbered by clothes as every other animal in there. With the Austin Powers theme tune blaring in the background we ran round and round, pausing every now and again to read the humorous signs the zoo had put up for us. 'Ants don't need pants, and neither do you,' I read as I completed lap one. 'Elephants swim without trunks,' I spotted on lap two. And my favourite: 'Ever seen a bear in a bra? Exactly!'

Giddy from giggling for two kilometres, I headed back to the changing room.

So what did my summer of naked running teach me about nudity? In all honesty, I came to pretty much the same conclusion Bart did: it isn't something to get your knickers in a twist about. Running naked taught me to stop worrying about what my body looks like and instead be grateful for what it can do. Our bodies are beautiful and nothing to be ashamed of, and naked running celebrates that fact like nothing else. Talking as the girl who used to perform Houdini-esque contortions under a towel to avoid anyone getting a glimpse of exposed skin in the school changing rooms, this was a huge revelation for me. Like Bart, I haven't done another nude race since, not because I feel self-conscious or squeamish but because, as he rightly said, there just aren't a lot of opportunities to run naked (though www.nuderuns.com lists a few if you're nudey-curious). But some words of warning if you are, by any chance, tempted to try it: do remember that if you have big boobs it's probably best avoided... and that you do so without Vaseline at your own risk!

'Why we love running naked'

I've run naked races simply because I thought it would be hilarious to say I'd done them. I was very self-conscious at first but once you've started it's no different to any other race and you want to compete (I came second last year). My friends think I'm mad, but hey, at 54, when you're slowing down, signing up for a naked race means you're guaranteed to finish much higher up in the field. What I found most challenging was going up to receive my prize starkers!

Tim, 54, Kent, England

Being naked is natural – I don't consider it an 'interest'. What I like about naked running is the feeling of freedom. It's much the same as running in clothes: a powerful mix of achievement and 'please let this be over soon'. My teenage kids do not approve, but then it's their job not to. My wider family are proud of me, in a one-eyebrow-raised kind of way.

Emma Bourgeois, 46, London, England

'The taxi driver slammed on his brakes when he heard where I was heading'

In my thirty-ninth year, wanting to keep life interesting, I decided to step outside my comfort zone at least once a month. Among other things I tried a stand-up-comedy course, a mud run and tone-deaf-to-tuneful singing lessons (I'm still rubbish). I was researching obstacle races online when I spotted a naked swim. I mentioned it at work as I thought it was funny. One of my 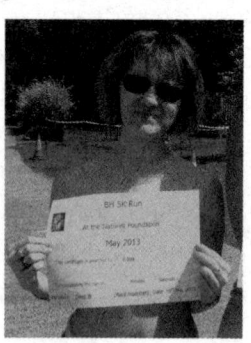 colleagues then told me of a 5K naked run in Orpington, so I looked it up. Bingo – there was my new thing to do that month.

The train got me to Orpington station in plenty of time but the taxi driver hadn't heard of the address so he managed to get a bit lost. Eventually, I had to confess exactly where I needed to go – and why.

It was just as well I was wearing my seatbelt as he slammed on the brakes to turn round and get a good look at me. No, I hadn't taken my clothes off yet, but maybe he thought I had!

It felt really weird undressing in the loos – I was ghostly white and wished I'd recently been on holiday to pick up a suntan. But when we started running I nearly forgot we were naked because Lisa and I were chatting so much.

I still find naturism a hard concept to get my head round but I'm quite a spiritual person so I can see that perhaps the absence of clothes allows you to get to know someone's soul rather than having preconceived ideas about them based on how they dress.

The strangest part of the day? Standing naked apart from a pair of trainers and having the race director's wife draw a race number on my arm with lipstick. I'm not sure I'd run naked again, but I'd definitely encourage others to do it!

Kim Neal, 41, London, England

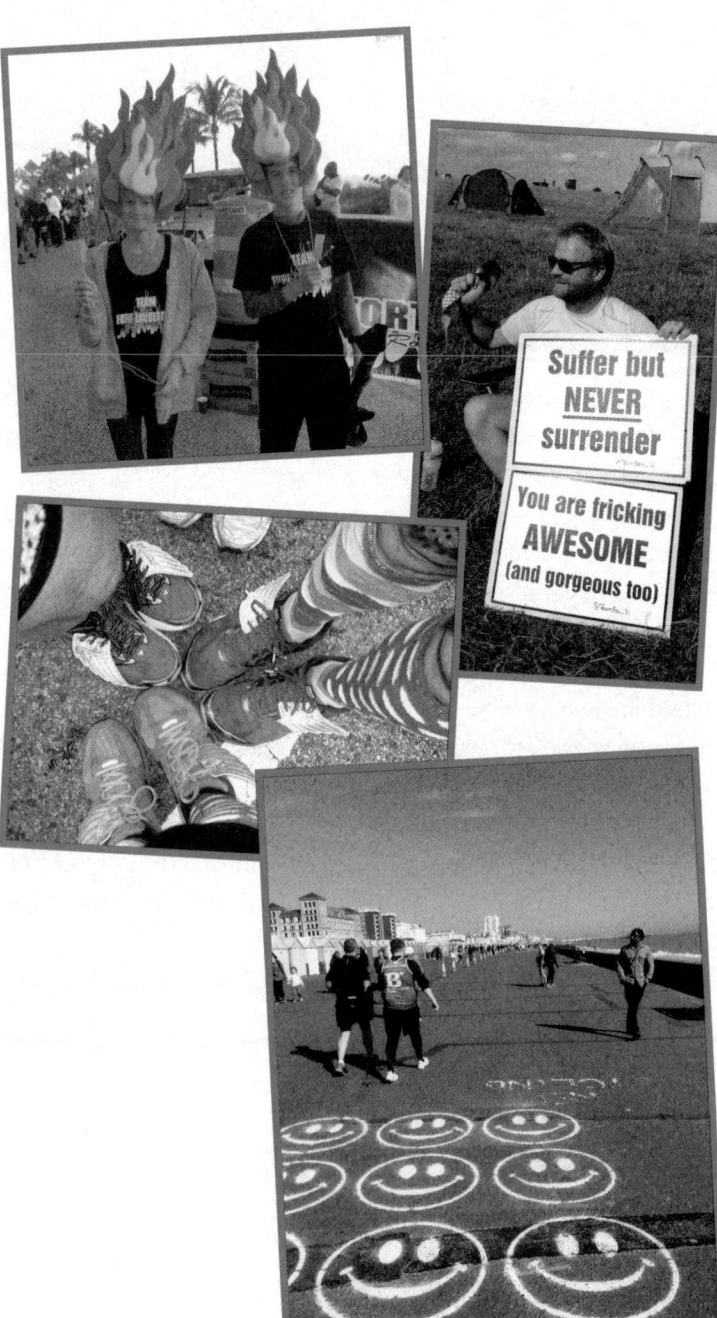

Chapter 10

What I can teach you about running

> " You don't learn to walk by following rules. You learn by doing, and by falling over "
>
> Richard Branson

So what would I say to those happy to take advice from a woman who spends half her running life dodging the Grim Sweeper? Truthfully all the wisdom I've amassed can probably be summarised by the following: 'Vaseline *everywhere*. Chat-run/walk. Have fun. Chocolate when you need an energy boost. Graciously accept medal. Whoop (out loud). Sleep wearing medal. Repeat.'

But on deeper reflection there are a few other gems I can share with you, starting with some of the mistaken beliefs that have held people back from running – I hope you have fun seeing how many you too have held over the years.

MISTAKEN RUNNING BELIEFS

Mistake #1 'Someone needs to give me permission to become a runner'

Something that delighted me about running when I first started was that for once I didn't have to get anyone's permission. Unlike in my day job where I had to get my editor to approve every feature I wanted to write, choosing to run was stunningly simple. I just walked into the Definition Delicatessen, decided how I'd like to start redefining myself, and then reached up and pulled down the jar labelled 'Runner'. Mainly because it sounded a whole lot more appealing than 'Sofa Slob'. Yes, I'd have to pay the price required (the training, a few sacrificial toenails, etc), but that decision didn't require anyone's approval – except my own. Later on I'd drop by the Deli again and pick up the packets labelled 'Marathon Runner', 'Trailrunner', 'Triathlete', 'Ultrarunner' and '100-mile Walker'. The labels you desire may be 'Run/walker', '5K finisher', 'Healthier', '100 parkrunner' or 'Sub-four-hour marathoner' – it doesn't matter what you decide on, just make sure that whatever's inside truly floats your boat.

Also remember that every time you put one foot in front of the other at a pace anything faster than a walk, you are a runner. The forums where certain people take it upon themselves to define whether someone qualifies as a jogger or a runner based on their minute-per-mile pace utterly enrage me. Bart Yasso once wrote: 'I often hear someone say "I'm not a real runner". We are all real runners, some just run faster than others. I never met a fake runner.' Trust the man, he's run a helluva lot more competitive races (over 1,000 and counting) than some of those self-appointed Jogging Judges.

Mistake #2 'I must love running to run'

I met Victor Vella while walking backwards up the Acropolis to stretch my legs the day after the Athens Classic Marathon. Victor told me that he'd done 22 marathons in the four years he'd been running.

'Wow, that's impressive!' I said. 'Athens was my twenty-second too, but I've taken *eleven* years to get there.' And then Victor said something that astounded me: 'I don't really like running,' he confessed, 'but I've heard it keeps you young and healthy, so I *force* myself to do it. The only days I don't go running is when it's raining. So every day I wake up and pray for rain!' (Just so you know, he's now trying to break world records for his age group in ultramarathons.) Meeting Victor made me feel a whole lot better about the amount of running-hating I do. When I stop running long enough to think about it, it always seems my old friend running and I have a love-hate relationship. I've wrestled with this 'running rocks, running sucks' debate my entire running career and I'll probably go to my grave flip-flopping between the two opposing views. For every time that running is pure undiluted joy, when I'm running next to someone lovely and just floating almost effortlessly along, there's a time that running is so freaking hard it's like bashing my head against a brick wall. I'll be honest, at those times it's only enjoyable when it stops. And that's OK. Because if you add up all the amazing moments (even if most of them occur only *after* you've stopped) and then compare them to the number of hellish ones, the former outstrip the latter 1,000 to one. Because the combination of actually running and the feeling of having run make you feel more alive, more connected, more brimful of happiness than any other activity on earth. Trust me, as a part-time running-hater, I know what I'm talking about!

Mistake #3 'Everything – including my kit – has to be perfect before I start running'

If I'd waited until I was slim, fit or fast enough, or had the time to train, I'd still be waiting to start running. If you insist on perfection before you embark on any running journey your dreams are going to turn into mirages. And don't think you need the cash to splash on all the latest kit either. I can always spot newbie marathoners as they're the ones with nutrition belts bristling with gels and protein bars, placing their faith in their kit rather than their training. Money can't buy perseverance, or speed. Yes, I've been known to spend two days' salary on vitamin pills and supplements and have bought a pricy Phiten titanium necklace just because World Record Holder Paula Radcliffe endorsed it, and yes, I used to spend £10 on blister plasters before every marathon before I discovered Vaseline between the toes works just as well. But I'm wiser now. I know that in order to start all you really need is a decent pair of trainers, trackpants and a T-shirt (and a sports bra if you're female) – and the simple desire to start.

Mistake #4 'The only way to measure my running success is by my speed'

I've come last in 20 marathons. But so far I've done 90 (and two 56-mile ultras). Does that make me a failure as a runner – or a runaway success? Running can be immensely pleasurable (at times!), so why do so many people try to get it over with as soon as they can? You never see anyone in the middle of an aromatherapy massage tapping their watch and saying: 'How much longer to go?' Yet many runners think that getting from point A to point B as speedily as possible is the *only* goal running has to offer. I happen to think differently. And surprisingly, two-time US Olympian Kara Goucher agrees with me: 'That's the thing about running: your greatest runs are rarely measured by racing success. They are the moments in time when running allows you to see how wonderful your life is.' Even Mahatma Gandhi knew what Kara and I are on about: 'There is more to life than increasing its speed,' the great man once said.

Although I'm full of admiration for the hares I know, who chase and achieve fast times and PBs (I am truly in awe of their ambition and commitment), there is a group of us tortoises who will never stand on a podium because race directors simply don't award prizes for 'most friends made', 'best scenery spotted' or 'most fun had'. Us slower runners have a lot more time to cover the same ground and so we get to savour all the subtle shades of every single race. We have time to smell and photograph the bluebells (as I did in the Bewl Water Marathon in Kent). We have time to laugh at a llama (as I did in the Geneva Marathon). We have time to swap the most unusual names we've ever heard of (as I did with India Sun in the Tucson Marathon). We have time to chuckle at the plump-as-a-partridge pheasants in a field waddling faster than we are (as I did in the Beauty and the Beast Marathon). We have time to sing Zulu praise songs led by a man playing the tambourine (as I did in the Paris Marathon). We have time to help others through a dark patch – or be helped by them. We have time to play. As Nic, an exuberant marathon virgin with whom I ran a 6h40 time in Brighton, put it: 'By taking longer we make sure we get maximum value for money!'

And as a new friend, Anya, whom I met in Jamaica's Reggae Marathon, reasoned: If you consider a marathon to be an endurance event, who shows more endurance – the runners who finish in under three hours or those of us who take more than six?

Mistake #5 'If it's this bad now it can only get worse'

When my sister was trying to persuade me to do the 91K Comrades Marathon she told me: 'It gets bad, but it never gets beyond bad.' Having done Comrades three times, I now know this to be true. Even the legendary ultrarunner Ann Trason, who's won some of the world's most challenging ultras (including Comrades twice), agrees: 'It hurts up to a point and then it doesn't get any worse.' Trust in this wisdom, write it on the back of your race number so you won't forget it, and don't let a fear of temporary pain put you off dashing after your dreams. Oh, and if all else fails, for pity's sake, walk!

Mistake #6 'There are limits'

There really, truly aren't any limits. When I first started running I wholeheartedly believed 2K was my limit, as that's the length of the route my Dad had mapped out for me. Then I did the Grand Prix Fun Run 5K at Kyalami motor-racing circuit and found out I could do 3K more than that. I used to think I could only do one marathon (two at most) per year, until I realised I could safely do eight in ten weeks. And I think I may have mentioned my new limit is 91K (56.5 miles) in one day. It really is true that the more you do, the more you can do. And interestingly, we've been doing this since time immemorial. No one told the hungry San hunters in the Kalahari Desert that they couldn't chase an antelope for miles until it collapsed. Someone obviously forgot to tell the Zulu fighters who fought against the British in South Africa that running 96K (60 miles) on the same day as going into battle, as they frequently did, was impossible. And American ultrarunner Dean Karnazes, who can run for three days and nights without stopping, obviously didn't attend the briefing either. My all-time favourite running expression is probably the following: 'Running is 90 per cent mental – and the other ten per cent is mental, too.' By breaking any goal into bite-sized bits, anything is possible.

Mistake #7 'Running is boring'

Hello? Don't tell me you hadn't heard of chat-running before you read this book? Admittedly, I too found 'training' boring as I usually had to do it on my own and there was no medal waiting for me at the end. So I ditched training and found myself a wonderful running buddy called Belinda, whom I chat-run with for an hour twice a week (we call it 'passing the Talking Stick' and every run with her is a real hoot). Someone in the 100 Marathon Club once told me that the best training for a marathon is another marathon, and so I now, rather surprisingly, run a marathon almost every second weekend. That way I get to run with interesting new running companions on a regular basis, with a medal thrown in for good measure. Slow down to a conversational speed – whether in training or during a race – and I can promise you'll never have a dull moment.

If you're keen on staying fast, there are a host of things you can try to stop your running going stale: enter races that offer sensational snack opportunities; dedicate each mile to someone you love and remind yourself what they mean to you; try different running events like mud runs or obstacle races, or activities involving running such as orienteering or geocaching. Or become more mindful and pay attention to the beauty that surrounds you: crunching crinkling autumn leaves underfoot; the honeyed warmth of sunlight wrapping your skin in a soft shawl. Or pack your trainers and experience the soul of foreign countries through your soles. My dawn runs along the Malecón in Havana, through the vast temple-strewn Bagan plain in Myanmar (Burma) and in Death Valley, the lowest, driest, hottest area in North America, are some of my most treasured traveller's tales. It's up to you to put the fun back into every run.

Mistake #8 'It's OK to moan about running'

Actually, it's OK to moan *after* a race – just not during it. Heed the advice of Robert Louis Stevenson, the author of *Treasure Island*, who so sagely said: 'Keep your fears to yourself, but share your inspiration with others.' I deserved the nickname Moaner Lisa when I whined incessantly during the Istanbul Marathon, and for the first time ever a runner literally sprinted to get away from me (at least that's what it looked like!).

Staying positive proved to be a secret weapon when a friend asked me to take a marathon virgin, Nic, round the Brighton Marathon. 'She has major doubt as to whether she can do it,' she wrote. 'She'll be fine – but doesn't know it yet.' When I rendezvoused with Nic in the pre-race loo queue she told me she was terrified.

'I tend to be a glass-half-empty kind of person generally,' she said, 'and I'm *really* doubting myself.'

'Well, you can't be like that today!' I replied. 'You can whinge all you like when we've finished – but *during* the race it's our sacred task to keep each other positive. Today we are going to have a blast and make new friends along the way.'

Having Nic with me made it one of the best marathons I've run in years. She was just delightful: thanking *every* marshal and *every* supporter, cheering on *every* runner – and not the least bit embarrassed to do so. A highlight was sharing a sighting of the Queen with her – having done this race many times I knew that a certain supporter living in Hove always dressed up as Her Majesty in a headscarf, so I told Nic that she was waiting for us round the corner and she squealed with delight when she spotted her. At a time when my injured feet were starting to get me down, Nic was just the breath of fresh air I needed to remind me how much I truly adore running. A few days later she sent me this email: 'Having so much fun meant more to me than chasing a time. I heard of many people who did well time-wise but came away broken because they didn't get the time they wanted, whereas I have memories that'll never be erased. I have so much love for all the people we met and it changed my view on what matters and what doesn't.' The conclusion: positivity pays!

Mistake #9 'I can try new things on race day'

I've made this mistake innumerable times, and I've always, but always, come off second best. I decided to dress up as one half of the Tortoise and the Hare fable in the London Marathon one year, without trying out my costume in training first. It turned out to be the papier-mâché shell from hell, giving me unbearable backache virtually from mile one. I ran the Stockholm Marathon with a spanking new bumbag – and it sanded a patch of skin the size of a pitta bread off my stomach. I've had my arms almost sawn off by an untested T-shirt in the Eilat Desert Run half marathon in Israel. I drank the sinister sports drink at the 2004 Rome Marathon that saw a third of the field throwing up through the railings of the ancient ruins of the Forum. I've trialled eating dried apricots on the run during the Abingdon Marathon in Oxfordshire – and got a serious case of the runs as a result. And I listened to my Dad and stayed silent for the first half of my first Comrades, which made me so miserable I almost quit. Dear reader, do *not* try new things on race day. Just don't!

Mistake #10 'It's OK to keep running to myself'

I'll never forget the way my family, friends and colleagues shared their love of running with me, and encouraged me to join them. As the saying goes: 'Friends don't let friends drive... they make them run!'

Over the years my enthusiasm has rubbed off on many people I know, and sharing their successes has been one of running's biggest rewards. Take this email that I received from my friend Angela:

I did it... I did it... I did it... I did it... I did it... I did it! I'm so impressed with myself for doing my first half marathon yesterday, couldn't wait to tell you. I got myself into a bit of a state fretting about it and only had three hours' sleep the night before. The last 2.5 miles around the Cheltenham Racecourse were a killer. I walked a lot more than I wanted – and I had to queue for a wee for about four minutes – so I'm pretty impressed with my 2h04 time.

That email warmed my heart for a week. Over the years many people have unknowingly encouraged me, none more so than an anonymous 100 Marathon Club member I met at the Brighton Marathon back in 2010. When I revealed that I'd dearly love to join the Club, he asked me how many marathons I'd run.

'This is only my eighteenth, so I have a very long way to go,' I replied.

'Oh, we've *all* been there once!' he said encouragingly before disappearing into the distance.

The fact that he didn't scoff at my total, or try to put me off from emulating his achievement, gave me the courage to set my sights on joining the 100 Marathon Club myself. At first I saw it as a 15-year goal, but then, having done 12 marathons in 2012, I realised that if I pushed myself a little harder I could bring my timescale forward by ten years. And then in 2015 I readjusted my timescale once more. So now I'm aiming to say I've been there, done that and literally got the T-shirt around the time this book is published, a challenge that involves doing 25 marathons in a single year. And, having done 90 (and two ultras that also count), I'm well on my way to getting there, meaning that by the time I'm finished I'll have walked/run over 4,300 kilometres (2,672 miles), a distance equivalent to flying from London to Tehran in Iran. All thanks to the thousands of runners these past 17 years who've touched my life, patted me on the back, high-fived me or inspired me. You may even be one of them.

So if you see a runner in a 100 Marathon Club T-shirt and a flamingo hat, do slow down for a chat. I'm hoping it'll be me!

MAGICAL MARATHONS

There are some epic marathons and ultras I've done that will be on almost any runner's bucket list (London, New York City, Boston, Paris, Rome, Comrades) and I admit they're hard to beat as they boast huge numbers of participants, superb organisation and spectacular routes. And there are also ones I do every year (Beachy Head, Brighton, the Portsmouth Coastal Waterside and the Thames Meander) just because I've fallen in love with them and doing them repeatedly is the equivalent of hanging up a giant stocking for Father Christmas every 24 December – it's somehow comforting to turn them into an annual tradition. I'm also rather partial to UK events organised by Saxons, Vikings & Normans Marathons, White Star Running, TrailPlus and Enigma Running as their race directors seem to love fun, cake and funky or Frisbee-sized medals as much as I do. However, what follows is my selection of some of my favourite lesser-known marathons, each of which truly is 26.2 miles of pure joy...

Most hilly – and heavenly: Jerusalem Marathon (March)

'Come and run where the superheroes of all three religions have trod in the past,' said the flyer advertising this race. And despite its innumerable hills of truly biblical proportions I found myself loving running where Jesus, Mohammed and King David once walked. So much so that I've become positively evangelical about it. Yes, only a small section of the route runs through the cobbled Armenian Quarter of Jerusalem's Old City (the streets there are way too narrow for a large marathon field), but it's simply heavenly seeing the Mount of Olives and the Dome of the Rock glinting in the spring sunshine while being cheered on by Hasidic Jews dressed in distinctive black coats and hats. Bart Yasso called this 'the most brutal road race I've ever run,' so I'm chuffed to bits to call myself a two-time finisher.

Enter here: www.jerusalem-marathon.com

Most runner-friendly and fun:
Giant's Head Marathon (June)

Having been voted the UK's best marathon by *Runner's World* readers in 2014, in only the second year it was run, this horrendously hilly off-road race is full of quirky surprises such as a marshal dressed as a snowman and a naked farmer in a bath whose sole purpose is to cheekily cheer you on. Then there's the notorious Lovestation, which features party food such as biscuits, cake, crisps and watermelon… but also generous glugs of cider and cranberry-flavoured vodka. Finishers are awarded a bling-tastic medal featuring the Cerne Giant (aka 'Rude Man'), after whom the race is named – a 180-ft tall ancient naked figure that's cut into the nearby hillside. Afterwards, there's an utterly delicious slap-up meal and barn dance in the village hall, so you can compare notes and do-si-dos!

Enter here: www.whitestarrunning.co.uk

Most technical: Coniston Trail Marathon (June)

Boulders, a riverbed, sharp rocks, bridleways, cliff-edge footpaths – it's often described as the UK's most picturesque trail marathon, but it's also one of the most tricky underfoot. Comprising a single-lap loop around the shores of Coniston Water, one of the loveliest lakes in the Lake District, it takes in well-known selfie spots such as Tarn Hows (a mountain lake studded with waterlilies and set in woodland) and, after an energy-draining climb, gives you glorious views of the entire lake. Despite being so tough, it's beginner-friendly, too, and finishes at a very festive race village where you can listen to live music as you relive every scenic step.

Enter here: www.lakelandtrails.org

Most festive: Bacchus Marathon (September)

Modelled on France's infamous Marathon du Médoc, this funfest of a fancy-dress race, held at Denbies Wine Estate in Surrey, England, follows the same formula of mixing whining with wining: there are lots of tough old hills on the two-lap course, but then there are also scores of refreshment stations serving up snacks and award-winning wines. It's a favourite with 100 Marathon Club members, who sprint from aid station to aid station and then spend ten minutes at each one carousing, dancing and posing for photos. Don't miss the bare-chested gladiators (who obviously train all year just for the chance to show off their toned torsos) or the free hog-roast afterwards, which is just another chance to party some more.

Enter here: eventstolive.co.uk

Most scenic: Loch Ness Marathon (September)

'The roads will give you blisters; the mountains will give you goosebumps,' promise the organisers of this Scottish race that delivers the wow factor in spades (and I'm not even referring to the moment, mid-race, when I swear I saw a mysterious row of ripples in the lake). The scenery en route is quite simply breathtaking – alpine forests, heathered hillsides and bracken-covered mountains – and so is the course, which is a roller-coaster ride of ascents and descents. Special touches: free tea and coffee in the loo queue at the start – and a delicious hot meal at the finish. Tough but terrific.

Enter here: www.lochnessmarathon.com

Most moving: PZU Warsaw Marathon (September)

Visit the sobering Warsaw Uprising Museum and you can see footage of what the Polish capital looked like after the Second World War: the Nazis destroyed it so systematically that barely a brick was left standing. So to run a marathon through a city that has risen from the ashes to become such a vibrant place featuring futuristic skyscrapers and a lovingly restored thirteenth-century Old Town (now a UNESCO World Heritage Site) really is a tribute to the human spirit. The race starts and finishes at the iconic National Stadium, designed to look like a fluttering red-and-white Polish flag, and the flat route is designed to showcase most of the city's many sights, including lush and leafy Royal Lazienki Park with its 500 rare red squirrels. A very touching moment for me was running over one of the manhole covers that many resistance fighters and residents used to access the sewers and escape the Old Town during the Warsaw Uprising. Warm and welcoming, this is truly a world-class race.

Enter here: pzumaratonwarszawski.com/en

Most unexpectedly interesting venue:
Turin Marathon (October)

I don't just love this event because it's a race tradition to make as much fuss of those who come last as those who come first, though that certainly is very welcome. I love it because I'd never have visited Italy's former capital if I hadn't run a marathon there, and hence would've missed out on the fascinating Shroud Museum and the bizarre Cinema Museum housed in the Mole Antonelliana, described by our guidebook as 'a bishop's-hat dome, topped by a pagoda-like spire balancing on a mini Greek temple'. The flat course – there's only one very gentle slope between 25K and 28K (between 15.5 and 17.4 miles) – features a dramatic landscape encompassing a stretch along the mist-shrouded River Po. Plus there are sections through the surrounding villages where drummers and locals in traditional dress give you an avalanche of audible encouragement as you soak up the views of the snow-capped Alps.

Enter here: www.turinmarathon.it

Most unusual: Istanbul Marathon (November)

Being awoken by a muezzin on race day was just one moment of many that ensured that this race, the only marathon where you run on two continents, turned out to be a Turkish delight despite the fact that over half of the course is on an out-and-back flat highway. Cited at the crossroads of civilisations, Istanbul is one of the most buzzing cities in the world, and the section along the Bosphorus, with its multi-minaretted mosques, was magical. I ran my fiftieth marathon here and afterwards treated myself to a steam bath and massage in a traditional Turkish hammam, followed by a sandwich made with fish served up straight out of the Golden Horn from a gaily painted boat next to the Galata Bridge. It's customary to eat your sarnie with a side order of gherkins and cabbage in pink pickle juice – handily, the latter is proven to reduce post-workout muscle cramps.

Enter here: www.istanbulmarathon.org

Most authentic: Athens Classic Marathon (November)
A pilgrimage to the place where it all began just has to be a must-do on every marathoner's list. Admittedly the route isn't going to dazzle you – but the finish in the horseshoe-shaped Panathenaic Stadium most definitely will, and not just because it's clad in gleaming white marble. This stadium was the venue for the first modern-day Olympic Games, and it's utterly amazing to run into it just like Spyridon Louis, the Greek water-carrier who won the first Olympic marathon way back in 1896. It's said to be the hardest championship-quality course in existence, as the first 30K (18.6 miles) are all uphill, but the townspeople who come out to cheer you on – and hand out olive branches, a symbol of both peace and victory – make it a very moving experience.

Enter here: www.athensauthenticmarathon.gr

Most glamorous: French Riviera
Marathon Nice-Cannes (November)

Yes, I liked the red-carpet finish. And yes, I loved the sun-drenched views of Antibes that have been immortalised by Matisse and Picasso. And of course I adored the glamour of running in Brigitte Bardot's former stamping ground. But what I rated most highly about this A-list event is the way it's run around two bays, so you get the unique satisfaction of seeing exactly how far you've come – and how far you still have to go. Just don't get caught, like I did one year, licking sweat off your arm (as my friend Bridget had told me top runners do when they're in need of salt) in full view of a whole restaurant of *al fresco* diners and bemused waiters. The wonderfully warm weather in November, when the rest of Europe is just starting to get chilly, is yet another reason why Nice (to Cannes) is really rather nice!

Enter here: www.marathon06.com

'What running means to me'

When I approached well-known runners from around the world, many of whom have competed in the Olympics, won marathons, broken records and become legends, to contribute to my book, I asked them to put into words what role running has played in their lives. I expected most of them to talk only about the glory of breasting the finishing tape and their delight at standing on the winner's podium. However, the contributions I received surprised me because not one of these famous runners talked solely about those things. What they did refer to instead was how emotionally healing running is, how it makes them feel incredibly alive, the friends they've made, the freedom it brings. I was amazed and excited to discover that the über-achievers and gazelles at the front (whom I seldom, if ever, get to meet) aren't all that different to us plodders at the back (whom I do, all the time).

Running is my life – I still run every day, no one can take it away from me. Sure I wanted to be the best in the world, but my second goal was just to enjoy it! Some people wake up and immediately need a cup of tea or coffee to get going – not me, I just put on my clothes and go for a run. Every day starts from that point. I often run–walk if I'm tired, and just go out for longer. Provided you walk with passion and strength, like you have a mission, it's fine to walk. Getting out and being active is all that really matters. I love what running does for your body, and how good it feels while you're doing it. I also love the freedom of running: I grew up in Kenya and have moved back there so I go running in the middle of nowhere, where no one can bother me.

Lornah Kiplagat, Kenyan-born multiple World Champion and three-time Olympian

'Friendship' is what means most to me as a runner. Long after the cheers have died down, the prize money has been spent, and the newspaper headlines forgotten, the most enduring part of running is the friendships that are formed. Thanks to the common bond of running these friendships endure, and they are forged and solidified all around the world. They are such special friendships because runners are generally warm, welcoming people who share a passion for running, this most special human ability.

Bruce Fordyce, legendary South African nine-time winner of the Comrades Marathon

I hate it. No, seriously, I do. I hate not being able to breathe and I hate feeling like an old buffalo being made to dance for tourists, dragging my body round the park. In fact I wouldn't really call it running, what I do. It's more of a shuffle. I hate it when it rains or when a hundred faster runners pass me twice on the same run. But... I also love it. Because I still can't believe I'm capable of it. That someone like *me* can actually run two or three or, on one occasion, *ten* kilometres. I care nothing for PBs. I just aim to finish. And despite my love/hate relationship with running, I honestly don't think I'll ever stop. Because afterwards I feel on top of the world and I never, ever, ever regret it! It also means I can bury my face in trifle afterwards and just suck it all up in a glorious calorie-reimbursement fest!

**Ruth Jones, newbie runner (aka Nessa
in the British hit comedy series *Gavin & Stacey*)**

Running is my lifestyle. I view it in the same way I do brushing my teeth or eating breakfast. Running is my best friend. It is always there: rain, snow or sunshine. The longer I do it the more comfortable I am with it. I love the fact that I don't dread it. I've worked hard not to make it a chore. I've seen so many people say they *have* to run ten miles today. I look at it like I *get* to run ten miles today. I am so grateful for the fact that I can still run. I am also blessed that I can run. Never, never take it for granted.

**American Pam Reed, the first woman to become
the overall winner of the Badwater Ultramarathon**

What running means to me has changed over the years. It used to be all about finding ways to run faster and be a 'better' runner. Everything was about commitment and drive. Being married to a two-time Olympian marathon runner (Liz Yelling) and having a double European cross-country champion as a sister (Hayley Yelling) simply reinforced that. To be honest, I frequently found running painful and frustrating, punctuated by the occasional high of a performance peak. So what's changed? Running still means a lot to me but success in running now means something quite different: it's all about long-term health, enjoyment, participation – and time for myself (something you don't get much of with three young children!). Nowadays I'm rarely bothered about the pace I run at and more focused on where I'm running or whom I'm running with.

Martin Yelling, former England international athlete, endurance coach and founder of the Marathon Talk podcast and the physical-activity challenge Jantastic

I will always run. I run to test myself. I run to know that my limits are not where I thought they were. I run to see beautiful places, to get off the beaten track, to explore and have adventures. I run to see the changing seasons, to splash through puddles, or feel the sun on my face. I run to feel alive.

Chrissie Wellington, British triathlete and four-time World Ironman Champion

I started running because I was totally useless at everything else. I swim like a rock and have no ball sense. In gym classes at school we had to do a lot of gymnastics but I was so uncoordinated that I just stayed at the back of the line and never did anything. Everything changed when it came to running. It was, and still is, the only place I feel truly at peace with myself. It is my reset point in life. A lot of people look back into their past and have a reset point where life was OK and they felt OK. I find that in my running: every day I reset my spiritual and emotional self as well as physically finding my place in this world. Running is not about the run, but about living beyond mortality.

Zola Budd Pieterse, South African two-time Olympian

Running is freedom. It's as simple as that. These days we spend our lives being bombarded by emails, phone calls, constant demands. Head out on a run and, with each footfall, you delete an email; go for a run, and slowly but surely, everything slips back into perspective in our crazy, busy lives. The rewards are huge. There's the personal challenge; there's the camaraderie/buzz of a big race; there's the fabulous crowd support; there's also the fact that runners are, without exception, lovely, interesting, friendly people. But I must admit I'm also a sucker for that beautiful, job-done physical tiredness that wraps you up when you get back home after a long run. If I haven't had a run, my head buzzes with work hassles the moment it hits the pillow. If I've had a run, it's lights out, over and out. Nothing beats it!

Phil Hewitt, British author of *Keep on Running* and runner of 30 marathons in 12 different countries

I've been running since the late 1970s and have frequently been asked why we runners run. Perhaps because running is now so popular that it has crossed the barriers of both social class and international borders, someone once suggested to me that we run because it's become trendy to do so! They're wrong! The running boom originated because running doesn't have complicated rules, you can do it at any time, wherever you like, for as long as you like – and it's free. And, at least while you're actually doing it, you're your own boss, isn't that wonderful? Personally, I love running alone: I enjoy taking advantage of those little moments when there's nobody around and my mind is set free to clean up my own thoughts. But above all I enjoy how my body manages the physical challenge the road provides. My many years of experience tell me that running has nothing to do with wanting to be trendy, but has everything to do with simply falling in love with it.

Paco Borao, president of the Association of International Marathons and Distance Races (AIMS)

Running has been the greatest teacher in my life. Even as a little girl it taught me the joy of exploring the unknown – not just unknown places but my own limits, and I quickly learned that I could go further and faster than I'd ever thought possible! Even though I grew up on a farm where I could roam freely, running exposed me to a whole new world. It gave me the chance to make up my own rules: I could decide how fast, how far and where I wanted to run. It made me feel free and happy.

Elana Meyer, South African 1992 Olympic 10,000m silver medallist

In the workshops I teach I often talk about how we constantly edit ourselves to create a version of ourselves others will find acceptable. We're born whole, but spend our entire lives butchering ourselves down until we're a smaller version of ourselves. I believe running is one way to restore us to our 100-per-cent selves because it gives us a permission slip to be the playful, juicy, mischievous selves we were as children, before this editing process had taken place. Just think of kids at play: they run everywhere. Running isn't something they *have* to do, it's something they do instinctively, and enjoy doing, no matter how good they are at it. As adults, running gives us the gift of doing what we like doing – and there's no greater gift than that. And when it comes to choosing running challenges, let excitement be your compass. If you get excited about running fast, by all means speed up. But if running slowly and connecting with others and your surroundings does it for you, who says you can't make up your own rules and give yourself first prize for that?

Jamie Catto, singer/songwriter, founding member of British dance music supergroup Faithless

Some people run for charity, some for health. Me? I basically run for cheesecake, and cider, and chocolate, and all the treats I like to consume. Running for me is a hot, sweaty, nasty, hard activity during which I spend 95 per cent of the time staring at the ground ten feet in front of me wondering when I can stop and thinking 'Please legs, don't trip over'. I hate running. But I enjoy having done it and I like the rewards it brings (see the above list!). I often spend the tail-end of ultraruns daydreaming about what my food reward will be. I envy those who glide around looking at the world thinking 'Isn't this wonderful?' But that's not me. For me it's about the random people you meet out in the wilds or the runners you see week after week, often like-minded souls who share a love of running, I mean cake...

Traviss Willcox, chairman of the UK 100 Marathon Club and veteran of 357 marathons and 32 100-milers

Over the years, the reasons why I run have changed. In the past, running was a way to prove I could go faster and further than others. Right now, running is a pleasurable pastime that keeps me fit and healthy while bringing me into contact with some of the nicest people on this planet – parkrunners! I've used running to get closer to someone I wanted a deeper relationship with and I've used it to keep away from someone I no longer had time for. The one constant throughout my life has been that I use it to manage my mental well-being: it's the best antidote to stress I've ever known. When times are tough, when things just don't make sense, running delivers its biggest personal reward.

Paul Sinton-Hewitt, British founder of parkrun

Running is something I've done my entire adult life, and over the past 35 years it's had many definitions and purposes: it meant a college scholarship, a ticket to travelling the world, financial rewards, personal records. After the birth of my first child it developed a new purpose by becoming my 'happy pill', a way for me to stabilise my moods, to feel healthy, to manage my weight. I often say that running is like a maths equation – input versus output – the more I put into it, the more I get out. The role that running currently takes on in my life is 'social': running is when I can break away from the hustle of the day to meet my female friends to talk about our kids, our lives and to plan our future. Throughout the years the meaning of my running has changed but it is still my dearest companion.

Lisa Rainsberger, the last American woman to have won the Boston Marathon (in 1985), and two-time winner of the Chicago Marathon

When I was younger, running was training: I was a competitive canoeist and we ran to get fast. Now running is an escape: it gives me headspace; it's where I come up with creative ideas; it's what I do when I've got a problem to solve. I never listen to music and rarely time myself — this is time to step away from technology and listen to the birds singing and leaves rustling. I always head off-road if I can; it makes me feel connected to nature. I love that! When I go to events, it's all about the community. I don't care whom I beat or who beats me. When you've been overtaken by a pantomime horse in the London Marathon you stop worrying about things like that. I like to smile and wave and enjoy. Sometimes I get emotional and shed a tear. I am not quite sure why!

Danielle Sellwood, British co-founder of www.sportsister.com

Running's meaning has changed throughout my life. Now, at the age of 45, running is pure pleasure, my mistress, my muse. When I run I burst through the film of anxiety and overthinking that separates me from the stream of life. I am an animal. Free in myself and with others. There are no obligations on a run, no phone calls to pick up, no emails to return, no information to keep up with. It's playtime. I run how I feel. I'll race you if I fancy it. I'll always say hello. On train journeys when I see fields in the distance I imagine myself running through them. My trainers call me constantly. My skimpy shorts are a never-ending invitation. There is fun to be had in the forest. A parallel universe where all is simultaneously still and in motion. Running is my compass. My illicit thrill. My anchor. I've run today. Can you tell?

Paul Tonkinson, stand-up comedian and
***Runner's World* UK columnist**

Staying in shape was a big motivating factor for me when I started to run at 19. But quickly, running meant more to me than that; it changed the way I thought about my body for ever. I was a chubby child and hated PE, and when I hit my teens I became incredibly self-conscious and started dieting. I ate less and less, until I was skipping meals, lying to my parents about what I ate and losing weight dramatically. Thankfully, my parents noticed before too much physical damage was done, but my relationships with eating and my body were wrecked. When I started running longer distances in my late teens and early 20s, feeling the air rush into my lungs and my heart pumping blood to my hard-working muscles, I was amazed by the body I'd taken for granted and abused. I don't always love the way my body looks now, but through running I appreciate what it's able to do. My diet is far from perfect, but I would never skip a meal again – my running and my health mean too much to me.

Liz Hufton, editor of UK *Women's Running* magazine

T-SHIRT SLOGANS THAT HAVE MADE ME SMILE

Running was invented so water would taste good

I'll be over here doing what you say is impossible

Always be yourself.
Unless you can be a runner.
Then always be a runner

Slow runners make faster runners look good.
You're welcome

There will come a day when I cannot do this.
Today is not that day

'I really regret that run,' said no one. Ever

I have to keep going... I parked at the finish

First or last... it's still the same finish line

Success comes in a can, not a cannot

Pain is inevitable. Suffering is optional

Inhale confidence, exhale doubt

Last is the slowest winner

Last but having a blast!

YOU KNOW YOU'RE A REAL RUNNER WHEN...

- Ninety per cent of your laundry contains Lycra – and most of your running tops have holes in them (from pinning on race numbers)

- Frozen peas are not a foodstuff but an essential part of your first-aid kit

- You're convinced it's totally normal to talk to random strangers – just as long as they're wearing a race number

- You have your own name on most of your T-shirts, not a fashion designer's

- You air-kiss your friends not because you're being pretentious but because you don't want to get sweat on their face

- You sniff your T-shirt after training to smell how hard you've run

- You have a whole drawer in your kitchen dedicated to your gel and sports drink collection

The part of you that aches most after a race is your hand – all that high-fiving

Massage means only one thing to you: pain

You know the location of every bush, pub and public toilet within a 5-mile radius of your house

You think black is the new pink when it comes to the colour of your toenails

You don't wait for a doctor to measure your heart rate

Your friends have stopped asking you 'Are you still running?'

You've converted half of your friends into runners

You know that all marathons are exactly the same distance… and that all ultras aren't

A CRASH COURSE IN RUNNING-SPEAK

Every sport has its unique set of terms and trivia, so here's a quick quiz you can use to learn the lingo and brush up your running knowledge.

1. Which moustachioed runner, who was the Race Director of the London Marathon until 2012, and who always ran in red socks, sued a telephone-directory-enquiries company for caricaturing his likeness – and then gatecrashed its launch party?

2. In which city was the women's world marathon record set, by whom, in what year and in what time?

3. What movie character, who was depicted running up a flight of steps at the Philadelphia Museum of Art, did more for the city's image than 'anyone since Benjamin Franklin', according to Dick Doran, the City Commerce Director at the time?

4. What is the occupation and nationality of the runner who wrote *What I Talk About When I Talk About Running*?

5. What is a negative split?

6. The World Marathon Majors are six marathons boasting an international elite field that also have a mass field completing the same course and are regarded among the

best in the world. The World Marathon Majors offer a $1 million prize purse that's split equally between the top male and female marathoners in the world. Non-elite runners who have completed all six can order a special certificate. Can you name the six marathons?

7   Which marathon club's rules stipulate that to gain entry at the very least you need to have done either two marathons in 16 days or three in 90 days (the highest level of membership, Titanium, requires doing 52-plus marathons or running marathons in 20 countries in 365 days)?

8   It sounds like a derogatory term but what does the word *ugali* actually mean?

9   On which marathon course have ten world records been set (seven male and three female), making it the fastest in the world?

10   In which film does a bearded runner run across America – and invent the yellow smiley-faced logo along the way?

11   What is the name of Europe's oldest marathon and in which country is it held?

12   What does the term 'you just got chicked' mean?

13   How many of the following running acronyms can you decipher? DFL; DNF; DNS; DOMS; LSD; PB; PR; PW; WR

14 Should the term 'chip time' have you reaching for the ketchup? And if not, why not?

15 Which legendary British runner, a two-time Olympic 1,500m champion whose middle name is Newbold, said (while pointing to his head): 'The nine inches right here; set it straight and you can beat anybody in the world.'

16 What is the name of the legendary town in Kenya where 25 world champions, four Olympic gold medallists, Paula Radcliffe and Mo Farah have all trained? Its name is a local corruption of 'Hill Ten'.

17 What is the name of the world's largest running race with 64,000 runners, and where does it take place?

18 Do you need to say 'Excuse me!' after doing a fartlek? And if not, why not?

19 Which kitchen appliance belonging to his wife did Oregon-based track coach Bill Bowerman, a co-founder of Nike, famously ruin when developing the Nike Moon trainer?

20 Which marathon club boasts that eight times more people have climbed Everest than have done what its members have to do to gain full membership?

21 How many seconds per mile will losing 5 lb of weight shave off your time?

ANSWERS

1. Dave Bedford, who broke the 10,000m world record in 1973. 2. London, Paula Radcliffe, 13 April 2003, in a time of 2:15:25. 3. Rocky Balboa played by Sylvester Stallone in the movie *Rocky*. 4. Author Haruki Murakami is Japanese. 5. When you run the second half of a race faster than the first. 6. New York City, Chicago, London, Boston, Berlin and Tokyo. 7. Marathon Maniacs. 8. It's the maize porridge favoured by Kenyan elite athletes. 9. Berlin. 10. *Forrest Gump*. 11. The Košice Peace Marathon held in Slovakia. 12. That you've been passed by a woman during a race. 13. DFL: Dead f***ing last; DNF: Did not finish; DNS: Did not start; DOMS: Delayed onset muscle soreness (it normally peaks about 48 hours after a particularly intense or long run); LSD: no, not a reference to hallucinatory drugs, it's an abbreviation for 'long, slow distance', which refers to running longer distances at an easy pace; PB: Personal best; PR: Personal record (more common in America); PW: Personal worst; WR: World record. 14. No, it's the actual amount of time it takes a runner to go from the start of a race to the finish line, so called because it's a timing technology that involves attaching a computer chip inside a little plastic casing to your trainers (or having a computer chip in a strip on the back of your race number). Also known as your 'net time'. It's the counterpart to your 'gun time', which is the amount of time between the start gun going off and you crossing the finish line. In big races your gun time can be up to 20 minutes slower than your chip time. 15. Sebastian Coe. 16. Iten. 17. The GöteborgsVarvet Half Marathon in Gothenburg, Sweden. 18. No, the term means 'speed play' in Swedish and simply involves mixing periods of slow and fast running. 19. A waffle iron. 20. UK 100 Marathon Club. 21. Ten seconds.

'What I wish I'd known before I started'

It seems I'm not alone in having had a lot to learn about this running malarkey. From the body benefits of walk-running to the importance of wearing a fresh pair of running tights, here a host of runners share their hard-won wisdom...

I was a cyclist before I decided to run across Canada dressed as the comic-book superhero The Flash, a distance of 5,000 miles (8,000 kilometres), and so knew nothing about what to expect. It was a good job that once I started running I found I had a love for it, as this coast-to-coast challenge involved running the equivalent of 200 marathons in 300 days in temperatures ranging from minus 40°C to plus 40°C! I found the first 50 marathons a struggle as it took a while for my body to adapt, but after that I realised running was natural, something we're supposed to do. I was amazed by the fact that us humans can just keep on running – there's nothing that can stop us from continually plodding away. We really were born to run. I don't wish I'd known anything before I started, actually, because in a weird way being naive and having no clue as to what I was getting myself into was precisely what gave me enough courage to do it.

Jamie McDonald, British trans-Canadian runner, adventurer and part-time superhero

Someone could've told me that runners do things differently. We're not like most people, that's for sure. I've been training since I was nine – that's 31 years as a runner – and when you've been brought up on running, you tend to mix with lots of other runners. That's the life – and the customs that come with it – you get used to. Since retiring from being an elite athlete I've started to have a more 'normal' lifestyle, mixing with real people, and it is only now that I've come to realise that dashing off to wee in any roadside flora you may come across isn't normal, nor is relieving yourself behind a wall, as I've done due to nerves and inadequate loo provision at all too many foreign races. Oh, and I wish I'd known that spitting while running (let alone snot shots!) isn't ladylike!

Liz Yelling, two-time British Olympian and former training partner to Paula Radcliffe

During my first few years of running, I wish I'd known that, far from slowing you down, taking 30-second walk breaks every few minutes right from the start of a race can actually result in faster times and fewer injuries. I also wish that some doctor had told me what the research shows: that runners have fewer orthopaedic issues as they age, so we really don't have to worry about knackering our knees like everyone says we do!

US Olympian Jeff Galloway, coach to over a million runners through his 29 books and Run Walk Run Training Groups

I wish I'd known that you're still a runner even if you don't do races and gun for PBs. I'm happiest when I just head out the door without a plan of how far or how fast I'm going to run. But occasionally I give in to the voice in my head that says, 'Real runners do races and PBs', and end up signing up for an event and abandoning my rambling, meditative runs for speed sessions and ticking off miles. My last half marathon taught me a valuable lesson. I was determined to do it in under two hours and, as I followed the training programme, running gradually morphed from a pleasure to a pressure, and my runs became another thing to add to my to-do list. On race day I achieved the time I wanted, but I injured my knee and couldn't run for three months afterwards. I turned running from something that nurtured me into something that caused me stress and damaged my body. Loads of runners thrive on doing races and beating their times, and that's right for them. What I wish I'd known before I started is that I am not one of those runners, and I never will be, but actually, that's OK.

Sally 'The Running Guru' Brown, Lisa's marathon inspiration, author of *Live Longer: Your Whole Health Route to Longer Life*

I wish I'd known that running would give me superpowers! That I'd become better at time management; organising my day to fit running in between work, children and everything else. That if I was tired or lazy then a quick run would power up the batteries and propel me into productivity. That I'd grow my self-esteem, enlarge my friends list, start cooking super-healthy food and rarely get ill. I've even started wearing (running) tights — although so far I haven't got a Wonder Woman cloak! I had no idea how useful running was and ponder all those wasted hours before I discovered my hidden powers. I hope you find yours, too.

Juliet McGrattan, GP, *Women's Running* UK contributor and author

I wish I'd known something! All I did know on 5 January 1994 was that I needed to go for a run as I'd reached a very unhappy place in my life and had become nicotine and alcohol dependent. Luckily, I made a lottery-winning selection of choices in training, mileage and running shoes that meant I could teach myself to run, injury free, and fall in love with the simple art of running. Twenty-one years on and I'm still loving training for and running marathons. If anything, I wish I'd run more as there were occasions where I didn't make time or didn't have the courage to take part in certain races and running challenges. Hindsight is a marvellous thing but I wish I'd become a running coach years earlier as it's the people you meet along the way, and not one's own accomplishments, that make the running journey so interesting and fulfilling.

Rory Coleman, British veteran of 940 marathons, 235 ultramarathons and 12 Marathon des Sables, and holder of nine Guinness World Records

It's not about a time or a place – if you aim for those you'll fail the majority of the time. It's all about fun. If you enjoy your running, you'll train and race hard – good times and places will come from that. Your life needs to be balanced in every area. Don't do too much of anything: don't train too hard, work too hard, drink too hard. Make time for your family and have downtime. Sleep and rest well. Most events are actually completed in your head, so you need a clear mind to get through the challenge – and the training beforehand. Variety is key, too. Keep things fresh by doing different events that scare and challenge you. Try something new every year. Last year I took up flatwater kayaking; the year before I went on a navigation course. This year it's gliding. Simple is nearly always best: no GPS watches, no fancy kit, no energy products – just run and have fun.

Mark Bayliss, the eleventh person to complete the Enduroman Arch to Arc triathlon (running 87 miles from Marble Arch in London to Dover, swimming 21 miles across the English Channel, then cycling 180 miles to Paris)

When I started running as a 13-year-old I knew nothing. I am very grateful for that. Had I known girls were weaker, that training would mess with my hormones and turn me into a she-man with a moustache, that I would never have children because of the jiggling to my insides, that I would strain my heart, and that I would wear out my hips and end up in a wheelchair, I would never have entered my first race. By the time they told me all these ridiculous myths it was too late; I was already hooked. I am also glad that no one told me what a joy it was to be able to run for hours, that I would travel to exotic lands and meet amazing people, that I would run in the Olympics, that I would view every failure as a stepping stone to success, and above all that running would gradually strip away the illusion of the ego and reveal to me my True Self. Finding out all that for myself has been nothing short of delightful.

Lorraine Moller, four-time New Zealand Olympian and winner of the 1984 Boston Marathon

If you have an important race always grab a fresh pair of tights. What you don't want to do is grab Friday's training pair for a Saturday race only to discover a mystery bulge working its way down your inside thigh 6K into a 10K. Then at 8K trying to kick yesterday's rolled-up sweaty underpants out of the bottom of your tights' left foot hole. Not a good look and definitely not a tactic that's going to win you a gold medal. Trust me, I haven't got a single one.

Taylor Huggins, 42, 2h57 British marathoner

I've run since the age of five, as my army major Dad had us kids doing every sport imaginable including fencing (with swords, not the garden DIY type), always backed up with a fitness regime that included running. I ran until I was 20, then stopped exercise altogether when I discovered sex, drugs and sausage rolls. When I was in my early 30s my wife decided we should join a running club so we jumped on the race train and got crazily competitive. Then one day I realised that road racing was wearing me down. Constantly striving to improve was proving impossible. It was then that it dawned on me (duh!) that I lived in Dorset, which has amazing trails to run on. So I took up trail running and began to prioritise enjoyment over achievement. Since then I've raced along ancient paths, Roman roads and Saxon ox droves; I've watched cows give birth; I've stood in wonder in the centre of ancient stone circles and got lost, a lot. Eventually I started organising some amazing events with massive coastal vistas, through dark woods and beautiful rolling countryside. What I wish I'd known? That new friendships, fabulous scenery and fruit-flavoured vodka (yes, I serve it mid-race — why wait till afterwards?) can make a race just as memorable as any PB.

Andy Palmer, 48, race director,
White Star Running, Dorset, England

I used to think cross-training was just a bunch of runners getting angry: of course, some 30 years since I started running, I'm much more enlightened. When I was younger – and injured – I would sit in a darkened room and generally wallow in self-pity about why I couldn't run; it never occurred to me that there was LOOR (life outside of running). It was only after five years of continual knee and Achilles problems that I finally decided to 'get on my bike' – and I've never looked back since (I do look left and right, though, for fear of irate motorists). The benefits that cross-training has brought to my running have been enormous: running three or four times a week and supplementing this with a swim or bike ride have meant that, into my mid forties, I can still be competitive and, more importantly, enjoy my running. I might still get angry when I'm injured, but now I cross-train with a purpose.

David Castle, editorial director of *Men's Running*

I wish I'd known that we can run for the whole of life. I wish I'd known that every mile I ran as a teen and young man was a lifelong investment in my health, happiness, creativity and friendships. I never flinched when the street-corner gangs with their cigarettes jeered as we ran by on drizzly winter evenings, but I wish I'd known for sure (as I know now) that we were the ones who had it right. I wish I'd known that one day running would not be only for nerdy undersized boys like me, but would be the joy of millions. And I kind of wish I'd known that I'd meet my wife, Kathrine Switzer, through running, and one day would contribute a small bit to a book where she would write the Foreword.

Roger Robinson, Boston and New York masters record-breaker and author of *Running in Literature*

RUNNING BOOK RECOMMENDATIONS

There are innumerable running books out there, but these are some of my favourites.

Books on how to run

Nell McAndrew's Guide to Running by Nell McAndrew and Lucy Waterlow

Lore of Running by Tim Noakes

The Run-Walk-Run Method by Jeff Galloway

Make Sure of Your Comrades Medal by Don Oliver (Don's training schedules are available online at www.alsoranrunners.info)

Running Made Easy by Lisa Jackson and Susie Whalley

Real Women Run, Running Well and *Marathon & Half Marathon From Start to Finish* by Sam Murphy

Books on why we run

Marathon Woman by Kathrine Switzer

My Life on the Run by Bart Yasso

Born to Run by Christopher McDougall

26.2: Marathon Stories by Kathrine Switzer and Roger Robinson

The Runner's Guide to the Meaning of Life by Amby Burfoot

Dare to Run by Amit Sheth

The Courage to Start by John 'The Penguin' Bingham

Running Crazy by Helen Summer

Keep on Running by Phil Hewitt

USEFUL RESOURCES

Women's Running (UK) (womensrunninguk.co.uk)
and *Men's Running* (mensrunninguk.co.uk)
The UK's first and only running magazines just for women or men, they're packed with real-life inspiration, tips, tricks and marathon reviews.

Runner's World (www.runnersworld.com)
Its user-friendly website is indispensable for reading reviews of – and booking – UK races.

Association of International Marathons and
Distance Races (www.aimsworldrunning.org)
AIMS is an organisation consisting of more than 380 of the world's leading distance races, from over 100 countries and territories. Click on 'Calendar' to find international races.

Also Ran Runners (www.alsoranrunners.info)
The amazingly inspirational website run by Nikki Campbell that held my hand through all my Comrades Marathon training. I can't praise Nikki, or this site, enough.

www.marathontalk.com
Marathon Talk is the UK's most popular free weekly running podcast and is presented by former England international athlete Martin Yelling and Tom Williams (MD of parkrun UK).

UKRunChat (www.ukrunchat.co.uk)
An online community for runners of all abilities offering support, event info, product reviews and expert advice. There's a forum, Facebook page, race finder, YouTube channel and a twice-weekly live Twitter chat.

261 Fearless Movement (www.261Fearless.org)
A non-profit organisation and movement inspired by the 261 bib number that Kathrine Switzer wore in her first Boston Marathon. It empowers women globally by creating a non-competitive community and offering running clubs and training programmes.

www.sportsister.com
An online women's sports magazine that's packed with athlete interviews, race reviews and the latest women's sportswear reviews.

www.trekandrun.com
A fab website featuring race and gear reviews and a great YouTube channel.

Marathon Majors (www.worldmarathonmajors.com)
Information about six of the world's most incredible marathons; those who've run all of them get a special certificate.

This Girl Can (www.thisgirlcan.co.uk)

This Girl Can is a national campaign developed by Sport England that aims to get women and girls moving, regardless of shape, size and ability. It features a huge variety of different sports and has a fantastic section on running.

Parkrun (www.parkrun.org.uk)

Free, timed, sociable 5K events in parks around the UK taking place at 9am on Saturdays.

Fetcheveryone (www.fetcheveryone.com)

A website that enables runners to keep a record of their running, and gives everyone the chance to read about the activities of fellow runners.

The Fat Girls' Guide to Running (toofattorun.co.uk)

A running resource and support website specifically designed to cater for larger women.

Run Mummy Run (www.runmummyrun.co.uk)

An online running community for women (not just for mums!).

Lazy Girl Running (www.lazygirlrunning.com)
An inspirational blog by a woman who went from self-certified couch potato to marathon runner and running author.

100 Marathon Club (www.100marathonclub.org.uk)
A very useful site for planning races as it lists marathons and ultras throughout the world.

Marathon Maniacs (www.marathonmaniacs.com)
The minimum entry requirement is having run two marathons in 16 days or three in 90 days.

Marathon Globetrotters (www.marathonglobetrotters.org)
A free club for those who love to run abroad. To become a provisional member you need to have run marathons in five countries; full membership requires having run in more than ten countries.

Chapter 11

Your running record

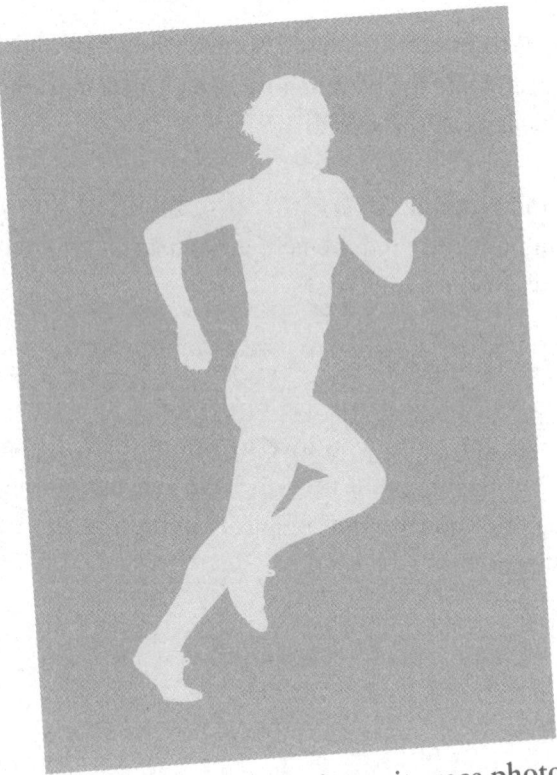

My favourite race photo

Once you've fallen in love with running you won't want to forget a single moment of it. Use these pages to create a record of your own treasured running memories, the snacks you've snaffled, the outfits you've worn, the people you've met and the places and races (OK, and the times, if you must!) you've run. Reviewing your accomplishments and goals will help you focus and spur you on when you're feeling discouraged.

RUNNING CURRICULUM VITAE

NAME _____

DATE WHEN STARTED RUNNING _____ / _____ / _____
AGE WHEN STARTED RUNNING _____

REASONS WHY I RUN

_____
_____
_____
_____
_____
_____
_____
_____
_____
_____

PROUDEST RUNNING MOMENTS

_____
_____
_____
_____
_____
_____
_____
_____
_____
_____
_____

'DREAMING BIG' GOALS
(races or places you want to run, time goals)

GOAL	DATE AIMED FOR	DATE ACHIEVED

MOST MEMORABLE RACES

FAVOURITE RUNNING MOTTO/MANTRA/RACE SIGN/ MOTIVATIONAL QUOTE

FUNNIEST RUNNING MOMENTS/
FAVOURITE STORIES HEARD ON RUNS

_____

_____

_____

_____

_____

_____

_____

_____

_____

_____

_____

FAVOURITE MEDALS/RACE T-SHIRTS

_____   _____

_____   _____

_____   _____

_____   _____

_____   _____

_____   _____

_____   _____

_____   _____

_____   _____

_____   _____

_____   _____

CHARITIES FUNDRAISED FOR AND AMOUNTS RAISED

CHARITY	AMOUNT RAISED

BIGGEST CHALLENGES OVERCOME IN RACES

RACES WITH THE BEST SNACKS/ENTERTAINMENT/ CROWD SUPPORT

_____   _____
_____   _____
_____   _____
_____   _____
_____   _____
_____   _____
_____   _____
_____   _____
_____   _____
_____   _____
_____   _____
_____   _____

FAVOURITE FANCY-DRESS OUTFITS

_____   _____
_____   _____
_____   _____
_____   _____
_____   _____
_____   _____
_____   _____
_____   _____
_____   _____
_____   _____
_____   _____

MOST BEAUTIFUL PLACES RUN IN

_____ _____
_____ _____
_____ _____
_____ _____
_____ _____
_____ _____
_____ _____
_____ _____
_____ _____
_____ _____
_____ _____

COUNTRIES I'VE RUN IN

_____ _____
_____ _____
_____ _____
_____ _____
_____ _____
_____ _____
_____ _____
_____ _____
_____ _____
_____ _____
_____ _____

CITIES I'VE RUN IN

_____   _____
_____   _____
_____   _____
_____   _____
_____   _____
_____   _____
_____   _____
_____   _____
_____   _____

MARATHON MAJORS COMPLETED

☐ London   ☐ Chicago
☐ New York City   ☐ Boston
☐ Berlin   ☐ Tokyo

FRIENDS I'VE MADE THROUGH RUNNING

_____   _____
_____   _____
_____   _____
_____   _____
_____   _____
_____   _____
_____   _____
_____   _____
_____   _____

MY PERSONAL BEST LIST

Best time for 5K/3.1 miles
Time_____ Date_____
Time_____ Date_____
Time_____ Date_____

Best time for 10K/6.2 miles
Time_____ Date_____
Time_____ Date_____
Time_____ Date_____

Best time for a half marathon (21.1K/13.1miles)
Time_____ Date_____
Time_____ Date_____
Time_____ Date_____

Best time for a marathon (42.2K/26.2miles)
Time_____ Date_____
Time_____ Date_____
Time_____ Date_____

Best time for an ultra
Time_____ Date_____
Time_____ Date_____
Time_____ Date_____

Best time for a triathlon
Time_____ Date_____
Time_____ Date_____
Time_____ Date_____

MY RACE RECORD

DATE OF RACE	DISTANCE	TERRAIN (TRACK, TRAIL, ROAD)

RACE NAME	TIME ACHIEVED

Acknowledgements

A huge thank you to...

... Claire Plimmer at Summersdale, who immediately greeted this book with great enthusiasm and fired the start gun for its publication.

... Debbie Chapman at Summersdale, who has run alongside me on this project, and whose encouragement and stamina have seen it through to the end. Our discussions and deliberations turned a potentially gruelling process into such a fun one that I was sorry to see it end. Thank you Debbie for your incredible eye for detail – and for always going the extra mile, even when it involved deleting about 400 exclamation marks! I'm in awe of your editing.

... Hamish Braid at Summersdale, who has crafted this book into a delightful depiction of my running journey. And to Angela Ryan (www.angelaryan.co.uk) who designed my book proposal and, as always, was a joy to work with. Also to Matthew Hams, whose delightful cover illustration perfectly expresses what this book is about.

... Ray Hamilton and Daniel Mersey, who have taken such care to make sure my book is typo- and error-free.

... photographers Victoria Adamson (photograph of Miette L Johnson), Rafa Babot (photograph of Lisa Jackson and

Kathrine Switzer in the Foreword), Eddie Macdonald (photograph of Christina Macdonald) and Team Bear Tri (bell-ringing supporter photograph on page 244) for letting me use your fabulous photos.

... Barbara Johnston, who started out as a fellow Comrade, but soon turned into my sounding board for this book. I've had so much fun editing this book with you and can't thank you enough for your input and inspiration. And to my running buddies Bridget Robinson, Belinda Carroll and Victoria Legge – thanks for almost always saying 'yes' when I suggest we enter yet another marathon and for being such a hoot on the road.

... my three 'unofficial' editors – Sarah Owen, Lucy Snow and Graham Williams – whose comments were invaluable. Many of my running friends also read my book proposal and drafts of this book and pointed out errors and omissions and made suggestions that have immeasurably improved it (any remaining mistakes are entirely my own fault). Sincere thanks to Megan Staley, Juliet McGrattan, Jamie Sawyer, Ian Beach, Bridget Robinson, Lize Lombard, Sally Brown, India Hesse, Penny Lovegrove, Cecy Montes, Tina Chantrey, Sue Atkinson, Nicola Kukuc, Helly Gilles and Pat Ivory. Special thanks to Jane Donovan, my editor on *Running Made Easy*, who continues to be my unofficial agent and cheerleader!

... the fabulously encouraging Kathrine Switzer, this book's Fairy Godmother, who bought me the little pot of glue that ensured my book proposal got written, and who helped ensure my Boston Marathon dream came true. With a woman like that in my corner, how could I possibly fail?

… Elizabeth Hufton, David Castle, Christina Macdonald and Danielle Sellwood – for allowing me to become the World's Slowest Marathon Correspondent (I can't imagine many editors would've shown the trust in me that you have). And to my utterly amazing English teachers – Jean Holmes, Gillian Hearn, Jenny Janisch and Verna Brown – who fostered a love of writing and reading in me that is one of life's greatest pleasures. Your passion and encouragement sowed the seeds for this book.

… all the wonderful runners who've shared their stories with me, both the ones I've included in this book and those I haven't. You have put many smiles (and a few tears) into the miles. Thanks too to all the well-known runners who were so generous with their contributions to Chapter 10 – you continue to inspire me in many different ways. Also to all my family and friends who've put up with my running evangelism and haven't seen me for months due to this book.

… all the members of the 100 Marathon Club who've made me green with envy while encouraging me to join them! Special thanks to Traviss Willcox, Roger Biggs and Rachel Smith for their support (including brownies). And to everyone at Striders of Croydon – I may be a ghost member but I know I'll always get a warm welcome when I do turn up.

… race directors the world over who've welcomed me to their races, many of whom have given me early starts (and late finishes) to ensure I got my medals. Also to all the many unsung heroes – the aid station volunteers, marshals and baggage bus personnel (whom my friend Megan Staley described as 'an inspiration, as are all the people who volunteer, getting water/ Powerade/gels tossed on them, after waking up before dawn to set up their tables and staying to clean up the mess we toss behind!'). Without you there would be no races to love.

… my beloved husband Graham Williams, who has run alongside me in the journey of life for 30 years, and who has done all the cooking, cleaning, shopping, sewing, ironing and housework for many years in order to give me time to write. You are amazing in every way – I just wish you didn't put up such a fight every time I suggest we do a marathon together.

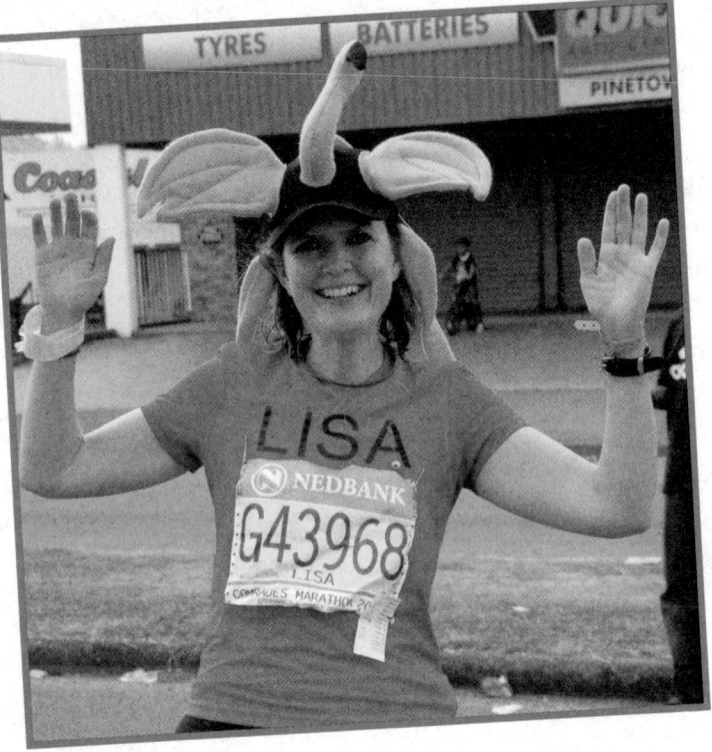

About the Author

Despite growing up in running-loving South Africa, it took health journalist-turned-hypnotherapist Lisa Jackson 31 years before she attempted her first marathon in 1999. The experience transformed the fitness-phobe into a running evangelist and inspired her to co-write *Running Made Easy*, which became Britain's best-selling beginners' running book, and which is still encouraging its readers (more than 100,000 at the last count) to give walk/running a go.

Now a Contributing Editor at *Women's Running*, Lisa also regularly writes for *Men's Running* and Sportsister.com. As the self-styled 'World's Slowest Marathon Correspondent', she has donned fancy dress to cover races in cities as diverse as Jerusalem, Boston, Durban, Istanbul, New York, Paris and Athens. Though Lisa's a wannabe member of the 100 Marathon Club – and a veteran of 90 marathons and two 56-mile ultramarathons – she often comes last!

Lisa lives in Croydon, south London, with her super-supportive husband Graham, who has run 27 marathons and two ultramarathons almost entirely against his will.

Contact Lisa if you enjoyed this book – or want to try hypnosis to boost your motivation. If *Your Pace Or Mine?* has inspired you to run for a minute, a mile or do a marathon or ultra, Lisa would love to hear from you. Drop her a line at quiet.medicine@gmail.com and she may even end up including you in a future book or magazine article. Lisa also offers hypnotherapy sessions for fitness motivation – visit www.quiet-medicine.co.uk for more information.

Have you enjoyed this book?
If so, why not write a review on your favourite website?

If you're interested in finding out more about our books,
find us on Facebook at Summersdale Publishers and
follow us on Twitter at @Summersdale.

Thanks very much for buying this Summersdale book.

www.summersdale.com